改訂6版

精神神経学用語集

日本精神神経学会・精神科用語検討委員会 編

2008

株式会社 新興医学出版社

目　　次

はじめに	*i*
精神科用語検討委員会	*iii*
凡　例	*iv*
本　文	*1*
外国語索引	*107*
外国語略語索引	*205*
解説用語	*207*
歴史用語	*210*
人名索引	*212*
参考資料	*215*
おわりに	*216*

はじめに

　平成13年（2001）8月、第12回WPA横浜大会の直前に、スティグマを助長しかねない（不適切な）用語として精神障害者およびその家族から呼称変更の要望が強く出されていた（精神）分裂病を行政用語としてのみならず学術用語としても統合失調症に変更することを本学会が公認した。その後、平成17年4月に厚生労働省が痴呆（症）の行政用語として「認知症」を用いるよう公示し、官報にも記載された。そこで、痴呆症の呼称変更問題に対し学術用語としてはどう対応すべきかが緊急の課題となり同年の第101回日本精神神経学会総会会期中の5月に当「精神科用語検討委員会」が設置された。委員会発足時担当理事であった関係で小生が委員長を務めることになった。さて、二つの用語の呼称変更のみならず、近年DSM-IV、ICD-10などの新しい診断基準が普及するなかで新しい精神科用語も急増する一方、本学会の旧「精神神経学用語集、1989」は20年近く改訂されないまま、新用語の大半が記載されていないため、また、平成17年4月発足した本学会の専門医制度ではケースレポートを書くことが要件になっているが、その際精神科専門用語は何を基準に書くかが問題となって、用語集の改訂への要望が急速に高まったと思われる。

　なお、本学会の用語集刊行の経緯は以下のとおりである。
1937年、「精神病学用語集」：林道倫委員長ら4名（精神神経学雑誌41巻4号）
1959年、「精神医学統一用語集」：島崎敏樹委員長ら4名（精神神経学雑誌61巻
　　　　号外）
1962年、「神経学統一用語集」：上田英雄委員長ら9名（精神神経学雑誌64巻号外）
1970年、「精神医学用語集」：加藤正明委員長ら8名
1989年、「精神神経学用語集」：加藤伸勝委員長ら11名
2008年、「精神神経学用語集・第6版」：松下昌雄委員長ら11名

　初年度は急を要する統合失調症および痴呆（症）関連用語の補遺の作成に当たった。統合失調症は精神科固有の用語なので、多くの関連用語のそれぞれについてかなり苦労したが、何とか「補遺」をまとめることができた。しかし、「痴呆（症）」は、神経内科、内科、老年科など他科にも跨る用語のため行政用語としての「認知症」が先行、流布してしまったが、学術用語としてどう扱ったらよいかとなると議論百出してまとまらず、本委員会は平成17年11月に評議員に対し、痴呆（症）に替わる学術用語として適切な用語は何か、という設問で4案｛下記の（1）～（4）｝を提示してアンケート調査を実施した。その結果は以下のとおりであった。

＜アンケート結果＞
アンケート用紙147通を発送、回収率71.9％であった。
　　（1）認知症（44.8％）
　　（2）認知衰弱症（または失知症）（略用語：認知症）（24.8％）
　　（3）失知症（17.1％）
　　（4）「痴呆症」のまま（12.4％）
　　（5）その他（1.0％）

　なお、そのほか具体的提案として、「認知能力減退症（略用語：認知症）」、「器質性認知機能障害」、「知忘症」、「知呆症」、「知的老化症」、「衰知症」などの提案があった。その結果を踏まえ委員会で議論し、(1)と(2)に絞って決をとったところほぼ半数ずつであったので、補遺作成のため取りあえずの学術用語として、「認知症」としてよいか、を理事会に諮問したところ結論的に、「認知症（痴呆[症]）」（仮）となった。その後特に新らしい意見はないが、平成18年度に入り、用語集・本文の検討に際し、それではいかにも複雑で判りにくいということになり、今回の第6版・委員会試案では二語を併記して「認知症，痴呆（症）」とした。

　学術用語は、内容を的確に表現し、できるだけ簡略で、一般的にも判りやすい用語が求められていると思うが、近年の社会情勢からスティグマを助長するような表現は避けるべきであるとなるとなかなか難しい。特に精神科の場合、問題用語としてすぐに「精神病」、「人格障害」などが頭に浮かぶが、一般社会と繋がりが深いのでやはり十分な配慮が必要と思われる。

　本用語集は学術的用語集なので、古い用語、不適切な表現となった用語であっても、歴史的に重要な用語は「歴史用語」として残した。また、多少の解説が必要と思われる用語には「解説用語」として簡略な解説をつけた。神経学用語は精神科と関連の深い用語のみに止めた（他に、日本神経学会の詳細な「神経学用語集・改訂第2版」(1993)がある）。また、精神科は社会との繋がりが深いので、ある程度精神科福祉関連用語も採用したが、それも幅を広げると際限がないので必要最小限度に止めた。

　本用語集の改訂に当たり、近年の社会の動きのスピードに合わせ本用語集も2〜3年に1度くらいは見直し、一部を修正するなり、補遺を出すなりすることが要請されていると感じたので、今後是非そのような配慮がなされるよう要請しておきたい。

　なお、参考とした書名は巻末にまとめて提示した。
　本委員会の構成は、次頁のとおりである。（平成20年4月）

精神科用語検討委員会

(2008年4月1日現在)

委員長
　松下　昌雄（帝京大学客員教授、社団法人社会福祉友の会西落合診療所（精神科）院長、日本精神保健福祉政策学会理事長（会長 故秋元波留夫）、JSPN評議員、前JSPN理事）

委　員
　内海　　健（帝京大学精神神経科学教室准教授）
　江口　重幸（財団法人精神医学研究所附属東京武蔵野病院・教育研究部長）
　鹿島　晴雄（慶應義塾大学精神神経科学教室主任教授、JSPN副理事長、当委員会担当理事）
　兼本　浩祐（愛知医科大学精神神経科主任教授）
　小山　善子（学校法人金城大学医療健康学部教授、前金沢大学大学院医学系研究科保健学専攻教授、JSPN評議員）
　鈴木　二郎（山王精神医学心理学研究所鈴泉クリニック所長、元東邦大学医学部精神神経科学教室主任教授、元JSPN理事長）
　中山　　宏（青梅成木台病院診療部長、元東京都立神経病院神経精神科部長）
　濱田　秀伯（群馬病院長、前慶應義塾大学医学部精神神経科准教授）
　福田　正人（群馬大学大学院医学系研究科神経精神医学准教授、JSPN評議員）

オブザーバー
　中根　　晃（横浜市西部地域療育センター児童精神科、日本自閉症スペクトラム学会会長、日本児童青年精神医学会名誉会員）

(注：JSPN＝社団法人日本精神神経学会)

凡　　例

【項目見出し及び配列】
1．配列は五十音順とした。
2．配列の原則は以下のとおり。
 1) 清音、濁音、半濁音、直音、拗音、撥音の別は無視した。
 2) 音引（ー）は無視する。
 3) 以上の結果、配列が同じになる場合は、清音、直音、音引なしをそれぞれ優先する。
3．見出しには、外国語を複数示す場合は、原則として英語、ドイツ語、フランス語、日本語、必要に応じてラテン語を付し、それぞれ（E）、（D）、（F）、（J）、（L）で表わした。但し、語のうしろに人名（その用語の提唱者等）がある場合はその人の国語を先頭に置いた。
4．事項のうち、ICD、PETなどの外国語の略語は纏めて外国語略語索引にABC順に配列した。
5．人名の表記
 1) 外国人名の場合、first nameは頭文字を「大文字」であらわした。
　〔例〕Eugen Bleuler → E. Bleuler
 2) 一人の氏名で原語に「-」がある場合は、「=」を入れた。
　〔例〕F. Fromm-Reichmann → F. Fromm=Reichmann
 3) 外国語人名の並列の場合は、ハイフン「-」を入れた。
　〔例〕レノックス-ガストー症候群
 4) 外国人名で、元のスペルが分かれている場合は、中グロ「・」を入れた。
　〔例〕ジル・ドゥ・ラ・トゥレット
 5) 日本人名は、日本語で「氏＋名」とした。
　〔例〕森田正馬
6．以下のことを示すために小括弧（ ）を用いた。
　別名、由来（提唱者名など）、略語、語のうち省略してもよい部分。
　〔例〕異食（症）、amnes(t)ic
7．入れ替えてもよい文字の場合は大括弧［ ］で示した。
　〔例〕disconnec[x]tion、投影［映］法
8．日本語として、あるいは日本語との対応関係について適切であるとは言い切れない語の肩にアステリクス2つ「**」をつけた。
　〔例〕説明と承諾**，cynanthropy **

9. 同義語あるいはほぼ同義の語については、併記または右矢印「→」によって関連を示した。
10. 解説が必要と思われる用語には（解説用語）をつけ、巻末に簡略な解説を施した。また、歴史的用語には（歴史用語）をつけ、巻末にまとめた。
11. 外国語略字（〔例〕ICD）および外国語索引、人名索引を巻末につけた。
12. 可能な限り用語の訳語として原則的に英語をつけた。
13. 神経学関連用語は右肩に、アステリスク1つ「*」をつけた。
14. 従来個人名の所有格として用いていたアポストロフィ「's」は、削除した。
〔例〕Broca's aphasia → Broca aphasia
15. カナとカナの間は、原則的に中グロ「・」とした。ただし、広く慣用されている用語は、個々に検討して2語間を詰めた。
〔例〕デイケア
16. 括弧が重なる場合は、大括弧の中は中括弧、中括弧の中は小括弧とした。
〔例〕［認知症｛痴呆（症）｝］
17. 参照語は、含意「⇒」で示した。
18. 併記した用語は、2語目以降の用語も別項目でも示した。

【本　文】

1) 用字・用語は常用漢字、新仮名遣いを原則としたが、専門用語、人名などは正字（略字、俗字以外）を用いた場合もある。また、近年新字体が慣用されている場合も意味内容からみて妥当と思われる場合は旧字体を用いた。
2) 年号は、西暦を用いた。

【参考資料】

参考資料は、巻末に一括して載せ、配列は書名の五十音順とし、それぞれ編者、著者または訳者等一名と、出版社、刊行年のみを示した。

以　上

あ

ICU症候群	intensive care unit syndrome（E）
アカシジア→静坐不能	
亜急性壊死性脳脊髄症（リー病）*	subacute necrotizing encephalo-myelopathy（Leigh disease）（E）
亜急性海綿状脳症*	subacute spongiform encephalopathy（SSE）（E）
亜急性硬化性全脳炎*	subacute sclerosing panencephalitis（SSPE）（E）
悪臭恐怖	dysosmophobia（E）
悪性症候群	neuroleptic malignant syndrome（E），syndrome malin（F）
悪魔憑き	demonomania（E）
悪夢	nightmare（E）
アゴニスト，作動物質［薬］	agonist（E）
亜昏迷	Substupor（D）
阿闍世コンプレックス	Ajase complex（古澤平作）（E）
アステリクシス*→姿勢保持困難*	
アスペルガー症候群	Asperger syndrome（E）
アダルトチルドレン	adult children（E）
圧縮	condensation（E），Verdichtung（D）
圧迫幻視	Druckvision（D）
アテトーゼ*	athetosis（E）
アドヒアランス	adherence（E）
アナルトリー→構音不能	
アフターケア	aftercare（E）
あぶら顔	oily face（E），Salbengesicht（D）
アヘン類	opioid（DSM-IV）（E）
── 依存	opioid dependence（E）
── 関連障害	opioid-related disorders（DSM-IV）（E）
── 使用障害	opioid use disorders（E）
── 中毒	opioid intoxication（E）
── 中毒せん妄	opioid intoxication delirium（E）

──誘発性障害	opioid-induced disorder（E）
──乱用	opioid abuse（E）
──離脱	opioid withdrawal（E）
アヘン類誘発性	opioid-induced（DSM-Ⅳ）（E）
──気分障害	opioid-induced mood disorders（E）
──睡眠障害	opioid-induced sleep disorders（E）
──性機能不全	opioid-induced sexual dysfunction（E）
──精神病性障害　幻覚を伴うもの／妄想を伴うもの	opioid-induced psychotic disorder with hallucinations/ with delusions（E）
アメンチア	Amentia（D）
アモク	amok（E）, Amok（D）
あるがまま	perceive reality as it is（E）
アルゴラグニー	algolagnia（E）
アルゴリズム	algorism（E）
アルコール	alcohol（E）
──依存（症）	alcohol dependence（E）
──患者匿名会	alcoholics anonymous（AA）（E）
──関連障害	alcohol-related disorders（E）
──幻覚症	alcoholic hallucinosis（E）
──症	alcoholism（E）, Alkoholismus（D）
──使用障害	alcohol use disorders（E）
──精神病	alcoholic psychosis（E）
──中毒	alcohol intoxication（E）
──中毒せん妄	alcohol intoxication delirium（E）
──てんかん	alcohol epilepsy（E）
──不耐性	alcoholic intolerance（E）
──乱用	alcohol abuse（E）
──離脱	alcohol withdrawal（E）
──離脱せん妄	alcoholic withdrawal delirium（E）
アルコール誘発性	alcohol-induced（DSM-Ⅳ）（E）
──気分障害	alcohol-induced mood disorders（E）
──持続性健忘障害	alcohol-induced persisting amnestic disorders（E）

——持続性認知［痴呆］症	alcohol-induced persisting dementia（E）
——障害	alcohol-induced disorders（E）
——睡眠障害	alcohol-induced sleep disorders（E）
——性機能不全	alcohol-induced sexual dysfunction（E）
——精神病性障害　幻覚を伴うもの／妄想を伴うもの	alcohol-induced psychotic disorders with hallucinations/ with delusions（E）
——不安障害	alcohol-induced anxiety disorders（E）
アルツハイマー型老年認知［痴呆］症	senile dementia of Alzheimer type（SDAT）（E）
アルツハイマー病	Alzheimer disease（E）
アルファ昏睡	alpha coma（E）
アルファ波	alpha wave（E）
アレキシシミア，アレキシサイミア　→失感情（言語）症	
アロヒリー*	allochiria（E）
暗示	suggestion（E，F）
暗示療法	suggestive therapy（E）
アンタゴニスト，拮抗物質（薬）	antagonist（E）
アントン症候群	Anton syndrome（E）
アンビバレンツ→両価性	
アンフェタミン	amphetamine（E）
——依存	amphetamine dependence（E）
——関連障害	amphetamine-related disorders（E）
——中毒	amphetamine intoxication（E）
——中毒せん妄	amphetamine intoxication delirium（E）
——使用障害	amphetamine use disorders（E）
——乱用	amphetamine abuse（E）
——離脱	amphetamine withdrawal（E）
アンフェタミン誘発性	amphetamine-induced（DSM-IV）

――気分障害	amphetamine-induced mood disorders（E）
――障害	amphetamine-induced disorders（E）
――睡眠障害	amphetamine-induced sleep disorders（E）
――性機能不全	amphetamine-induced sexual dysfunction（E）
――精神病性障害	amphetamine-induced psychotic disorders（E）
幻覚を伴うもの／妄想を伴うもの	with hallucinations/ with delusions（E）
アンモン角硬化	ammon horn sclerosis（E）
安楽死	euthanasia（E）

い

イェール・ブラウン強迫尺度	Yale-Brown Obsessive Compulsive Scale（Y-BOCS）（E）
域外幻覚	extracampine hallucination（E）
息止め発作	breath-holding spell（E）
医原神経症	iatrogenic neurosis（E）
医原性疾患	iatrogenic disease（E）
移行対象	transitional object（E）
意識	consciousness（E），Bewußtsein（D）
意識閾	Bewußtseinsschwelle（D）
意識狭窄（症）	Bewußtseinseinengung（D）
意識減損発作	seizure with impairment of consciousness（E）
意識混濁	clouding of consciousness（E），Bewußtseinstrübung（D），obnubilation（F）
意識障害	disturbance of consciousness（E），Bewußtseinsstörung（D），trouble de la conscience（F）
意識性	Bewußtheit（D）

意識喪失	loss of consciousness（E），Bewußtlosigkeit（D）
意識内容	Bewußtseinsinhalt（D）
意識変容	Bewußtseinsveränderung（D）
意識野	field of consciousness（E）
（易）刺激性	irritability（E），Reizbarkeit（D）
意志欠如	Willenslosigkeit（D）
意志欠如型（精神病質者）	Willenlose（Psychopathen）（K. Schneider）（D）
意志作用	Willensakt（D）
意志薄弱	Willensschwäche（D）
異常感覚	dysesthesia（E）
異常体感	abnorme Körpersensation（D）
異常酩酊	abnormer Rausch（D），abnormal drunkenness（E）
異食（症）	pica（L）
異性愛	heterosexuality（E）
異染性白質ジストロフィー*	metachromatic leukodystrophy（MLD）（E）
異層神経症	Fremdneurose（J. H. Schultz）（D）
依存	dependence（E），Abhängigkeit（D）
依存（性）パーソナリティ［人格］障害	dependent personality disorder（DSM-III）（E）
依存的	dependent, anaclitic（E）
依存抑うつ	anaclitic depression（R. Spitz）（E）
一次動因	primary drive（E）
一次妄想	primary delusion（E），primärer Wahn（D）
一次利得	primary gain（E）
一過性全（般）健忘	transient global amnesia（E）
一過性脳虚血発作*	transient ischemic attack（TIA）（E）
一級症状	Symptome 1. Ranges（K. Schneider）（D），first rank symptoms（E）
一側（性）失行，一側運動失行	unilateral apraxia（E）
遺伝子型	genotype（E）

遺伝素質	Erbanlage（D）
遺伝予後	Erbprognose（D）
イド→エス	
易怒性躁病	gereizte Manie, zornige Manie（D）
いなずま恐怖	keraunophobia（E）
遺尿（症）	enuresis（E）
犬神憑き	cynanthropy **（E）
猪瀬型肝脳疾患	hepatocerebral disease of Inose type（E）
EBM→エビデンス医学	
遺糞	encopresis（E）
イマーゴ	Imago（C. G. Jung）（D）
意味記憶	semantic memory（E）
意味健忘	semantic amnesia（E）
意味妄想	Bedeutungswahn（D）
イム	imu（E）, Imudo（D）
意欲減退	hypobulia（E）, Hypobulie（D）
意欲錯誤	parabulia（E）
意欲増進	hyperbulia（E）, Hyperbulie（D）
医療保護入院	admission for medical care and protection（E）
院外患者	outpatient（E）
因果関連	kausaler Zusammenhang（K. Jaspers）（D）
因果的説明	kausales Erklären（D）
飲酒試験	alcohol test（E）, Alkoholtrinkversuch（D）
インスティテューショナリズム→施設症	
インスリンショック療法	insulin-coma treatment（E）, Insulinkomabehandlung（M. Sakel）（D）, Insulinschocktherapie（D）
陰性幻覚	negative hallucination（E）, hallucination négative（F）
陰性症状	negative symptoms（E）

陰性症状評価尺度	Scale for the Assessment of Negative Symptoms（SANS）（E）
咽頭反射*	pharyngeal reflex（E）
院内寛解	intramural remission（E）
インフォームド・コンセント，説明と承諾	informed consent（E）
隠蔽記憶	screen memory（E），Deckerinnerung（S. Freud）（D）
韻律障害	dysprosody（E）

う

ウィスコンシンカード分類テスト	Wisconsin Card Sorting Test（WCST）（E）
ウィルソン病*	Wilson disease（E）
ウェクスラー児童用知能検査	Wechsler Intelligence Scale for Children（WISC，改訂版 WISC-R，3版 WISC III）（E）
ウェクスラー成人用知能検査	Wechsler Adult Intelligence Scale（WAIS，改訂版 WAIS-R，3版 WAIS III）（E）
ウェザニア（歴史用語）	vesania（E），vésanie（F）
ウェスト症候群	West syndrome（E）
ウェルニッケ失語	Wernicke aphasia（E）
ウェルニッケ脳症*	Wernicke encephalopathy（E）
迂遠	circumstantiality（E），Umständlichkeit（D）
ウシ海綿状脳症*	bovine spongiform encephalopathy（BSE）（E）
打ち消し→取り消し	
内田-クレペリン精神作業検査	Uchida-Kraepelinscher Rechentest（D）
うっ血乳頭*	choked disc, papilledema, papillary stasis（E），Stauungspapille（D）
うつ病⇒抑うつ	depression（E），Depression（D），dépression（F）
うつ病エピソード	depressive episode（E）

うつ病性仮性認知［痴呆］症	depressive pseudodementia（E）
うつ病性昏迷	depressive stupor（E）
うつ病性障害	depressive disorders（E）
瓜二つの錯覚	illusion des sosies（J. Capgras & J. Reboul-Lachaux）（F）
運動維持困難*，動作維持困難	motor impersistence（E）
運動過多（症）*	hyperkinesia(-sis)，hypercinesia(-sis)（E）
運動緩慢*	bradykinesia（E）
運動機能の特異的発達障害	specific developmental disorder of motor function（ICD-10）（E）
運動幻覚	kinesthetic hallucination（E）
運動減少（症）*	hypokinesia(-sis)，hypocinesia(-sis)（E）
運動失語（症）	motor aphasia（E）
運動失調*	ataxia（E）
運動常同	Bewegungsstereotypie（D）
運動心迫	Bewegungsdrang（D）
運動精神病	Motilitätspsychose（C. Wernicke）（D）
運動能力障害	motor skills disorder（DSM-IV）（E）
運動暴発	Bewegungssturm（D）
運動無視	motor neglect（E）
運命強迫	Schicksalszwang（S. Freud）（D）
運命分析	Schicksalsanalyse（L. Szondi）（D）

え

A型行動パターン	type A behavior pattern（E）
A群人格障害	personality disorder cluster A（DSM-III-R）（E）
エイズ認知症複合	AIDS dementia complex（E）
A-Tスプリット	A-T split（E）
鋭波	sharp wave（E）
エクムネジー→新規健忘	
エゴグラム	egogram（E）
壊死性脳炎*	necrotizing encephalitis（E）

エス	Es（D），id（E），ça（F）
エッシャー症候群	Asher syndrome（E）
エディプス・コンプレックス	Oedipus complex（E）
エネルギー・ポテンシャル減衰	Reduktion des energetischen Potentials（K. Conrad）（D）
エピソード記憶	episodic memory（E. Tulving）（E）
エビデンス医学，実証医学	evidence-based medicine（EBM）（E）
FTD-17	frontotemporal dementia and parkinsonism linked to chromosome 17（E）
MRI（磁気共鳴画像）	magnetic resonance imaging（E）
MRA（磁気共鳴血管造影）	magnetic resonance angiography（E）
MRS（磁気共鳴スペクトロスコピー）	(nuclear) magnetic resonance spectroscopy（E）
MSLT（睡眠潜時反復テスト）	multiple sleep latency test（E）
エレクトラ・コンプレックス	Electra complex（E）
遠隔記憶	remote memory（E）
鉛管様固縮［強剛，強直，硬直］*	lead-pipe rigidity（E）
演技（性）パーソナリティ［人格］障害	histrionic personality disorder（DSM-III）（E）
エングラム→記憶痕跡	
嚥下障害*	dysphagia（E）

お

応急入院	emergency hospitalization（E）
おうむ返し言葉	parrot-like speaking（E）
狼憑き	lycanthropy（E）
置き換え	displacement（E），Verschiebung（D）
汚言	coprolalia（E）
オセロ症候群	Othello syndrome（J. Todd & K. Dewhurst）（E）
おどけ（症）	clownism（E）
オペラント条件づけ	operant conditioning（E）
親虐待症候群	battered parents syndrome（E）
親指しゃぶり	thumb sucking（E）

折りたたみナイフ現象*	clasp-knife phenomenon（E）
オルガズム機能不全	orgasmic dysfunction（E）
音韻障害⇒発達（性）構音障害	phonological disorder（DSM-IV）（E）
音楽幻聴	musical hallucination（E）
音楽てんかん	musicolepsy（E）
音楽誘発性てんかん	musicogenic epilepsy（E）
音楽療法	music therapy（E）
音声（性）チック	vocal tic（E）
音素性錯語	phonemic paraphasia（E）
音連合	Klangassoziation（D）

か

外因好発型	exogene Prädilektionstypen（K. Bonhoeffer）（D），exogenous predilection type（E）
外因精神病	exogenous psychosis（E）
外因反応型	exogene Reaktionstypen（K. Bonhoeffer）（D），exogenous reaction type（E）
外界意識（精神）	Allopsyche（C. Wernicke）（D）
絵画統覚テスト	thematic apperception test（TAT）（E）
開眼失行*	apraxia of lid opening（E）
諧謔症，モリア⇒ふざけ症	moria（E）
外向	extraversion（E）
介護保険	long-term care insurance（E）
下意識	Unterbewußtsein（D）
外示記憶，顕在記憶	explicit memory（E）
解釈	interpretation（E），Deutung，Auslegung（D），interprétation（F）
解釈妄想（病）	délire d'interprétation（P. Sérieux & J. Capgras）（F）
外傷→心的外傷	
外傷後ストレス障害→心的外傷後ストレス障害	
外傷神経症	traumatic neurosis（E）

外傷性記憶	traumatic memory（E），souvenir traumatique（F）
外傷（性）てんかん	traumatic epilepsy（E）
外傷認知［痴呆］症	traumatic dementia（E）
解除反応，解放反応	abreaction（E）
回心	conversion（E），Bekehrung（D）
回心体験⇒回心	Bekehrungserlebnis（D），conversion experience（E）
解体	dissolution（H. Jackson）（E）
解体型統合失調症	disorganaized schizophrenia（E）
回転ドア現象	revolving door phenomenon（E）
回転（性）めまい*	vertigo，rotatory vertigo（E），Drehschwindel（D）
概日周期睡眠障害	circadian rhythm sleep disorder（E）
概日リズム，サーカディアンリズム ── 睡眠障害	circadian rhythm（E） circadian rhythm sleep disorder（E）
概念崩壊	Begriffszerfall（D）
回避（性）パーソナリティ［人格］障害	avoidant personality disorder（DSM-Ⅲ）（E）
快不快原則［原理］	Lust-Unlust-Prinzip（D）
回復記憶	recovered memory（E）
外来患者	outpatient（E）
外来現象	phénomène xénopatique（P. Guiraud）（F）
快楽原則［原理］	Lustprinzip（S. Freud）（D），pleasure principle（E）
快楽殺人	Lustmord（D）
快楽消失，アンヘドニア	anhedonia（E）
解離	dissociation（E，F）
解離性健忘⇒心因性健忘	dissociative amnesia（E）
解離性障害	dissociative disorder（E）
解離性同一性障害⇒多重人格性障害	dissociative identity disorder（DSM-Ⅳ）（E）
解離性遁走⇒心因性遁走	dissociative fugue（E）
解離ヒステリー	dissociative hysteria（E）

か

会話および言語の特異的発達障害	specific developmental disorders of speech and language（ICD-10）（E）
カウンセリング	counseling（E）
替え玉錯覚，フレゴリの錯覚	illusion de Frégoli（P. Courbon & G. Fail）（F）
加害恐怖	blaptophobia（E）
加害的被害者	persécuté persécuteur（F）
過覚醒	hyperarousal（E），Überwachheit（D）
（可）覚醒昏睡	coma vigil（F）
下顎反射*	jaw jerk（E）
過換気症侯群	hyperventilation syndrome（E）
鍵体験	Schlüsselerlebnis（E. Kretschmer）（D）
加虐性愛，サディズム	sadism（E）
可逆認知［痴呆］症	reversible dementia（E）
核間性眼筋麻痺*	internuclear ophthalmoplegia（E）
学習困難	learning difficulty（LD）（E）
学習障害（解説用語）	learning disability（LD）（E）
核上性眼筋麻痺*	supranuclear ophthalmoplegia（E）
覚性，覚性状態	vigilance（E）
覚醒アミン中毒	Weckaminvergiftung（D）
覚醒暗示	Wachsuggestion（D）
覚醒意識	Wachbewußtsein（D）
核性眼筋麻痺*	nuclear ophthalmoplegia（E）
覚醒［せい］剤精神病	amphetamine psychosis（E），Weckaminpsychose（D）
覚醒てんかん	Aufwachepilepsie（D. Janz）（D），awakening epilepsy（E）
覚醒発作	Wachanfall（D）
覚醒夢	Wachtraum（D）
学生無気力症，ステューデントアパシー	student apathy（E）
確認強迫	Kontrollzwang（D），checking compulsion（E）
学力の特異的発達障害	specific developmental disorders of scholastic skills（ICD-10 新訂版）（E）

下肢静止不能［むずむず脚］症候群	restless legs syndrome（E）
過書	hypergraphia（S. G. Waxman & N. Geschwind）（E）
過剰記憶→記憶増進	
寡症状性統合失調症	symptomarme Schizophrenie（D）
過剰適応	overadjustment（E）
臥床癖	clinomania（E），Bettsucht（D）
過食（症），大食（症）	bulimia（E）
過［狂］信型精神病質者，熱中［狂］型精神病質者	Fanatische（Psychopathen）（K. Schneider）（D）
仮性記憶，偽記憶	pseudomnesia（E）
仮性球麻痺*，偽性球麻痺*	pseudobulbar palsy（paralysis）（E）
仮性幻覚，偽幻覚	pseudohallucination（E）（F）
仮性認知［痴呆］症，偽（性）認知［痴呆］症	pseudodementia（E）
下層意志機制	hypobulischer Mechanismus（E. Kretschmer）（D）
画像失認	picture agnosia（E）
画像診断	diagnostic imaging（E）
画像性，形象性	Bildhaftigkeit（D）
下層知性機制	hyponoischer Mechanismus（E. Kretschmer）（D）
家族会	organization of the family with the mentally ill（E）
家族精神医学	family psychiatry（E）
家族否認妄想	family denial delusion（E）
家族分裂	family schism（E）
家族暴力	family violence（E）
加速歩行*	festinating gait，festination（E）
家族力動	family dynamics（E）
家族療法	family therapy（E）
過代償	overcompensation（E）
カタプレキシー→脱力発作	
カタルシス，浄化	catharsis（E）
カタレプシー，強硬症	catalepsy（E）

学校恐怖	school phobia（E）
渇酒癖	dipsomania（E）
葛藤	conflict（E）
家庭［内］暴力	home violence, domestic violence（DV）（E）
過敏情動性衰弱状態	hyperästhetisch-emotionaler Schwächezustand（K. Bonhoeffer）（D）
カフェイン中毒	caffeine intoxication（E）
カフェイン誘発性睡眠障害	caffeine-induced sleep disorder（E）
カフェイン誘発性不安障害	caffeine-induced anxiety disorder（E）
カプグラ症候群	Capgras syndrome（E）
雷恐怖	astraphobia（E）
過眠（症）	hypersomnia（E）
仮面うつ病	masked depression（E）, larvierte（maskierte）Depression（D）
仮面てんかん	masked epilepsy（E）
仮面様顔貌*	mask-like face, masked face（E）, Maskengesicht（D）
空の巣症候群	empty nest syndrome（E）
簡易精神症状評価尺度	Brief Psychiatric Rating Scale（BPRS）（E）
簡易精神療法, ブリーフ・サイコセラピー	brief psychotherapy（E）
寛解	remission（E）, Remission（D）
考え不精, 思考怠惰	Denkfaulheit（D）
感覚解離	sensory dissociation（E）
感覚過敏	hyperesthesia（E）
感覚記憶	sensory memory（E）, Sinnesgedächtnis（D）
感覚錯誤	Sinnestäuschung（D）
感覚失語（症）	sensory aphasia（E）
感覚遮断	sensory deprivation（E）
感覚消去*, 知覚消去	sensory extinction（E）
感覚対側逆転*→アロヒリー	

感覚鈍麻	hypesthesia（E）
眼球回転発作*	oculogyric crisis（E）
環境反応	situational reaction（E），Milieureaktion（D）
がん恐怖	carcinophobia（E）
環境療法	milieu therapy（E）
眼筋麻痺*	ophthalmoplegia（E）
関係妄想	delusion of reference（E），Beziehungswahn（D），délire de relation（F）
間欠性爆発性障害	intermittent explosive disorder（DSM-IV）（E）
喚語困難⇒語健忘	naming difficulty（E），Erschwerung der Wortfindung（D）
ガンサー症候群	Ganser syndrome（E）
ガンザーのもうろう状態	Ganserscher Dämmerzustand（D）
かんしゃく発作	temper tantrum（L）
患者クラブ	patient club（E）
患者自治会	patient council, patient government（E）
慣習犯罪者→常習犯罪者	
感情	feeling（E），Gefühl（D），sentiment（F）
感情移入	empathy（E），Einfühlen（D），Einfühlung（D）
感情移入的了解	einfühlendes Verstehen（D）
感情移入不能	Uneinfühlbarkeit（D）
感情失禁→情動失禁	
管状視野狭窄	tubular concentric contraction（E）
感情障害	affective disorder（ICD-10）（E）
季節性—	seasonal affective disorder（E）
混合性—	mixed affective disorder（E）
双極性—	bipolar affective disorder（ICD-10）（E）
感情精神病	Affektpsychose（D）
感情調節薬	thymoleptica（L）

感情鈍麻	Gefühlsabstumpfung (D), blunted affect (E)
感情病	affective illness (E)
感情表出	expressed emotion (EE) (E)
感情誘因性妄想	katathymer Wahn (D)
緩徐進行性失語（症）*	slowly progressive aphasia (E)
眼振*	nystagmus (E)
肝性脳症*	hepatic encephalopathy (E)
完全寛解	vollständige Remission (D), perfect remission (E)
感染症精神病	Infektionspsychose (D)
間代	clonus (E)
間代けいれん	clonic convulsion (E), klonischer Krampf (D)
鑑定留置	detention for psychiatric evidence (E)
観念（性）運動失行*	ideomotor apraxia (E)
観念（性）失行*	ideational apraxia (E)
観念貧困	Ideenarmut (D)
観念奔逸	flight of ideas (E) Ideenflucht (D)
観念連合	Ideenassoziation (D)
肝脳疾患*	hepatocerebral disease (E)
間脳症*	diencephalosis (E)
間脳症候群	diencephalic syndrome (E)
感応精神病	induced psychosis (E), induzierte Psychose (D)
感応性妄想性障害	induced delusional disorder (ICD-10) (E)
願望パラノイア	Wunschparanoia (D)
顔面失行*	facial apraxia (E)
顔面チック	facial tic (E), tic facial (F)
緘黙（症），無言（症）	mutism (E), Mutismus (D)
関与しながらの観察	participant observation (H. S. Sullivan) (E)
肝レンズ核変性症（ウィルソン病）*	hepatolenticular degeneration (Wilson disease) (E)

緩和医療	palliative medicine（E）
緩和ケア	palliative care（E）
緩和病棟	palliative care unit（E）

き

奇異反応	paradoxical reaction（E）
記憶	memory（E），Gedächtnis（D），mémoire（F）
記憶幻覚	Gedächtnishalluzination（D）
記憶減退	hypomnesia（E），Hypomnesie（D）
記憶痕跡，エングラム	memory trace（E），engram（E），Engramm（R. Semon）（D）
記憶錯誤	paramnesia（E）
記憶作用	mnemic function（E）
記憶障害	Gedächtnisstörung（D），dysmnesia（E）
記憶増進，過剰記憶	hypermnesia（E），Hypermnesie（D）
擬音語	onomatopoeia（E）
機会的同性愛	occasional homosexuality（E）
機会犯罪者	occasional criminal（E）
飢餓精神病	Inanitionspsychose（D）
器官愛	organ erotism（E）
器官言語	organ language（E）
器官神経症	Organneurose（D）
器官選択	Organwahl（D）
器官劣等性	organ inferiority（E），Organminderwertigkeit（A. Adler）（D）
偽記憶→仮性記憶	
危機介入	crisis intervention（E）
利き手	handedness（E）
利き脳	brainedness（E）
利き眼	eyedness（E）
既経験感	déjà éprouvé（F）
偽幻覚→仮性幻覚	

既視感	déjà vu（F）
気質	temperament（E）,
器質性	organic
——うつ病性障害	organic depressive disorder（E）
——解離性障害	organic dissociative disorder（E）
——気分（感情）障害	organic mood（affective）disorder（ICD-10）（E）
——緊張病性障害	organic catatonic disorder（ICD-10）（E）
——幻覚症	organic hallucinosis（ICD-10）（E）
——健忘症候群	organic amnesic syndrome（ICD-10）（E）
——混合性感情障害	organic mixed affective disorder（ICD-10）（E）
——情動不安定（無力性）障害	organic emotionally labile（asthenic）disorder（ICD-10）（E）
——精神障害	organic mental disorder（ICD-10）（E）
——双極性障害	organic bipolar affective disorder（ICD-10）（E）
——躁病性障害	organic manic disorder（ICD-10）（E）
——パーソナリティ［人格］障害	organic personality disorder（ICD-10）（E）
——不安障害	organic anxiety disorder（ICD-10）（E）
——妄想性（統合失調症様）障害	organic delusional（schizophrenia-like）disorder（ICD-10）（E）
器質精神症候群	organisches Psychosyndrom（E. Bleuler）（D）
器質精神病	organic psychosis（E）
器質性妄想状態	organic delusional state（E）
器質認知［痴呆］症	organic dementia（E）
器質力動説	organodynamisme（H. Ey）（F）
希死念慮	suicide idea（E）

記述精神医学	descriptive psychiatry（E）
偽神経症性統合失調症	pseudoneurotic schizophrenia（E）
擬人法，擬人化	personification（E）
帰責能力	Zurechnungsfähigkeit（D）
帰責無能力	Zurechnungsunfähigkeit（D）
季節うつ病	seasonal depression（E）
季節（性）感情障害	seasonal affective disorder（E）
偽相互性	pseudomutuality（L. Wynne）（E）
起訴前鑑定	psychiatric expertise before indictment（E）
既体験感	déjà vécu（F）
既知感	Bekanntheitsgefühl（D）
吃音	stuttering（E）Stottern（D）
狐憑き	alopecanthropia, fox possession（E）
基底気分	Grundstimung（D）
基底欠損	basic fault（M. Balint）（E）
基底抑うつ	Untergrunddepression（K. Schneider）（D）
祈禱精神病	Invokationspsychose（森田正馬）（D）
企図振戦*	intention tremor（E）
偽（性）認知［痴呆］症→仮性認知「痴呆」症	
記念日反応	anniversary reaction（E）
機能幻覚	functional hallucination（E）
気脳写	pneumoencephalography（E）
機能精神病	functional psychosis（E）
機能変遷	Funktionswandel（V. v. Weizsäcker）（D）
気晴らし食い→むちゃ食い	
忌避妄想	delusion of being avoided（E）
気分安定薬	mood stabilizer（E）
気分易変性	Stimmungslabilität（D）
気分エピソード	mood episode（E）
気分高揚	hyperthymia（E）
気分循環症	cyclothymia（E）

き

気分循環性障害	cyclothymic disorder（E）
気分（感情）障害	mood（affective）disorder（E）
一般身体疾患による―	due to general medical condition（E）
器質性―	organic（E）
持続性―	persistent（E）
精神作用物質誘発性―	substance-induced（E）
反復性―	recurrent（E）
気分沈滞	hypothymia（E）
気分倒錯	parathymia（E）
気分と調和した［に一致した］精神病症状	mood congruent psychotic features（E）
気分と調和しない［に一致しない］精神病症状	mood incongruent psychotic features（E）
気分変調（症）	dysthymia（E），Verstimmung（D）
気分変調性障害	dysthymic disorder（E）
気分変動型（精神病質者）	Stimmungslabile（Psychopathen）（K. Schneider）（D）
基本障害	Grundstörung（D）
基本症状	basic symptom（E）
基本的信頼	basic trust（E. H. Erikson）（E）
記銘力	impressibility（E），Merkfähigkeit（D）
記銘力低下	disturbance of memorization（E），Merkschwäche（D）
逆向健忘	retrograde amnesia（E）
逆説睡眠	paradoxical sleep（E）
虐待	abuse（E）
逆耐性現象	reverse tolerance phenomenon（E）
逆転移，対抗転移	counter-transference（E），Gegenübertragung（D），contre-transfert（F）
吸引反射*	sucking reflex（E）
嗅覚発作	olfactory seizure（E）
救急精神医学	emergency psychiatry（E）
求心性視野狭窄*	concentric contraction of visual field（E）

急性一過性精神病性障害	acute and transient psychotic disorder（ICD-10）（E）
急性錯乱	bouffée délirante（F）
急性錯乱状態	acute confusional state（E）
急性散在性脳脊髄炎＊	acute disseminated encephalomyelitis（ADEM）（E）
急性ジストニア［ジストニー］	acute dystonia（E）
急性ストレス障害	acute stress disorder（DSM-IV-TR）（E）
急性ストレス反応	acute stress reaction（ICD-10）（E）
急性多形性精神病性障害	acute polymorphic psychotic disorder（E）
急性中毒	acute intoxication（E）
急性アヘン中毒	acute opioid intoxication（E）
急性アルコール中毒	acute alcohol intoxication（E）
急性幻覚剤中毒	acute hallucinogen intoxication（E）
急性コカイン中毒	acute cocaine intoxication（E）
急性大麻中毒	acute cannabinoid intoxication（E）
急性ニコチン中毒	acute nicotine intoxication（E）
急性デリール	délire aigu（F）
急性統合失調症様精神病性障害	acute schizophrenia-like psychotic disorder（E）
急性脳症候群	acute brain syndrome（E）
急速眼球運動＊	rapid eye movement（E）
吸入剤	inhalant（E）
——依存	inhalant dependency（E）
——関連障害	inhalant-related disorder（E）
——使用障害	inhalant use disorder（E）
——誘発性障害	inhalant-induced disorder（E）
——乱用	inhalant abuse（E）
球麻痺＊	bulbar paralysis, bulbar palsy（E）
教育精神療法	psychagogics（E）
教育分析	didactic analysis（E）
共依存	co-dependency（E）

境界知能	borderline intellectual functioning（DSM-IV）（E）
境界（性）パーソナリティ［人格］構造	borderline personality organization（O. Kernberg）（E）
境界（性）パーソナリティ［人格］障害	borderline personality disorder（DSM-III）（E）
境界例	borderline case（E）
驚愕てんかん	startle epilepsy（E），Schreckepilepsie（D）
驚愕反応	startle reaction（E），Schreckreaktion（D）
共感	sympathy（E），Mitfühlen（D）
共感覚*	synesthesia（E）
共感性光覚*	photic synesthesia，photism（E）
強硬症→カタレプシー	
恐慌性障害→パニック障害	
きょうされん（元共同作業所全国連絡会）	Japan Association of Community Workshop for Disabled Persons（E）
共時性	synchronicity（C. G. Jung）（E）
郷愁反応	Heimwehrreaktion（D）
狂信型精神病質者	Fanatische（Psychopathen）（K. Schneider）（D）
狂信者	Fanatiker（D）
強制収容所症候群	Konzentrationslagersyndrome（D），concentration camp syndrome（E）
矯正精神医学	orthopsychiatry（E）
強制にぎり，強制把握*	forced grasping（E），Zwangsgreifen（D）
共生幼児精神病（歴史用語）	symbiotic infantile psychosis（M. Mahler）（E）
鏡像焦点	mirror foci（E）
鏡像段階	stade du miroir（J. Lacan）（F）
橋中心髄鞘崩壊［融解］*	central pontine myelinolysis（E）
協調（運動）*	coordination（E）
強直間代けいれん	tonic clonic convulsion（E）
強直間代発作	tonic clonic seizure（E）

強直けいれん	tonic convulsion（E）, tonischer Krampf（D）
強直発作	tonic seizure（E）
共同（性）注視*	conjugate gaze（E）
共同偏倚*	conjugate deviation of eyes（E）
強迫	obsession, compulsion（E）, Zwang（D）
強迫感情	Zwangsaffekt（D）
強迫観念	obsessive idea（E）, Zwangsidee（D）
強迫（性）緩慢	obsessive slowness（E）
強迫儀式	obsessional ritual（E）, Zwangszeremoniell（D）
強迫疑惑	Zwangsskrupel（D）
強迫行為	compulsive act（E）, Zwangshandlung（D）
強迫思考	Zwangsdenken（D）
強迫（性）障害	obsessive-compulsive disorder（E）
強迫神経症	Zwangsneurose（D）
強迫的飲水→心因性多飲（症）	
強迫泣き, 強制泣き*	forced weeping, forced crying（E）, Zwangsweinen（D）
強迫人	Anankast, Zwangsmensch（D）
強迫（性）パーソナリティ［人格］障害	compulsive personality disorder（DSM-Ⅲ）（E）
強迫表象	Zwangsvorstellung（D）
強迫欲動	Zwangstrieb（D）
強迫笑い, 強制笑い*	forced laughter, forced laughing（E）, Zwangslachen（D）
恐怖（症）	phobia（E）
恐怖症性不安障害	phobic anxiety disorder（ICD-10）（E）
共有精神病（性）障害⇒二人組精神病	shared psychotic disorder（DSM-Ⅳ-TR）（E）
強力性	sthenisch（D）
虚偽記憶（症候群）	false memory（syndrome）（E）
虚偽性障害	factitious disorder（DSM-Ⅲ）（E）

局在症状	local symptom （E）
局在論→大脳局在論	
棘徐波昏迷	spike-wave stupor （E）
棘徐波複合	spike-and-wave complex （E）
棘波	spike （E）
虚言	lying （E），Lügen （D），mensonge （F）
虚言症（癖）	mythomanie （E. Dupré）（F），mythomania （E）
虚言妄想	délire de fabulation （F）
拒食	food refusal （E），Nahrungsverweigerung （D）
去勢不安	castration anxiety （E），Kastrationsangst （D）
拒絶症	negativism （E）
巨脳症*	megalencephaly （E）
虚無妄想	nihilistischer Wahn （D）
疑惑狂（歴史用語）	folie de doute （F）
疑惑癖	Zweifelsucht （D）
筋感幻覚	Muskelsinnhalluzination （H. Cramer）（D）
筋緊張低下*	hypotonia （E）
近時記憶	recent memory （E）
筋収縮性頭痛*	muscle contraction headache （E）
近親相姦，近親姦	incest （E）
禁断現象	Abstinenzerscheinung （D）
禁断症状	Abstinenzsymptom （D）
禁断療法	Entziehungskur （D）
禁治産→被後見	
緊張性頚反射*	tonic neck reflex （E）
緊張性頭痛	tension headache （E）
緊張病	Katatonie （D），catatonia （E）
キンドリング	kindling （E）

クヴァード症候群，擬娩	couvade syndrome （E）

空間恐怖	space phobia（E）
空間体験	Raumerleben（D）
空気嚥下症，呑気症	aerophagia（E）
空虚感	sentiment du vide（P. Janet）（F）
空笑	leeres Lachen（D）
空想虚言	pseudologia phantastica（L）
空想作話	phantastic confabulation（E）
空想認知［痴呆］症	dementia phantasitica（L）
空想妄想（症）⇒虚言妄想	délire d'imagination（E. Dupré）（F）
クオリティ・オブ・ライフ→生活の質	
口とがらし反射*	snout reflex（E）
口運び傾向，口部傾向	oral tendency（E）
苦痛性愛→アルゴラグニー	
屈曲性対麻痺*	paraplegia in flexion（E）
国親権限	parens patriae power（E）
クライエント中心療法→来談者中心療法	
クライネ・レヴィン症候群	Kleine-Levin syndrome（E）
クラインフェルター症候群*	Klinefelter syndrome（E）
クラーヴス	clavus（L）
くらやみ恐怖	nyctophobia（E）
久里浜式アルコール依存症スクリーニングテスト	Kurihama Alcoholism Screening Test（KAST）（E）
グリーフ・セラピー	grief therapy（E）
クリューヴァー-ビューシー症候群	Klüver-Bucy syndrome（E）
クレチン病*	cretinism（E）
クレペリン病	Kraepelin disease（E），Kraepelinische Krankheit（D）
クレーン現象	crane phenomenon（E）
クロイツフェルト-ヤコブ病*	Creuzfeldt-Jakob disease（E）
群発自殺	suicide cluster（E）
群発頭痛*	cluster headache（E）
訓練療法	training therapy（E），Übungstherapie（D）

け

ケアマネージャー	care manager（E）
軽うつ（病，症）	Subdepression（D），mild depression（E）
経験的遺伝予後	empirische Erbprognose（D）
軽作業期（森田療法）	light work stage（Morita therapy）（E）
計算強迫	Zählzwang，Zahlenzwang（D）
計算癖	arithmomania（E）
痙縮*	spasticity（E）
芸術療法	art therapy（E）
形象凝集	Bildagglutination（D）
形象性→画像性	
痙性歩行*	spastic gait（E）
痙性麻痺*	spastic paralysis（E）
軽躁（病）	hypomania（E）
軽躁（病）エピソード	hypomanic episode（E）
軽佻者	Haltlose（E. Kraepelin）（D）
経頭蓋磁気刺激（法）	transcranial magnetic stimulation（TMS）（E）
系統的脱感作（法）	systematic desensitization（E）
軽度認知障害	mild cognitive impairment（MCI）（E）
鶏歩*	steppage gait（E）
傾眠	somnolence，drowsiness（E），Somnolenz（D）
けいれん	convulsion，spasm（E），Krampf（D）
けいれん発作	convulsive seizure（E），Krampfanfall（D），crise convulsive（F）
けいれん療法	convulsive therapy（E），Krampfbehandlung（D）
激越うつ病	agitierte Depression（D）
激励法	Protreptik（D）
ゲシュタルト機能	Gestaltfunktion（D）
ゲシュタルト変遷	Gestaltwandel（D）
ケース・マネジメント	case management（E）
血液脳関門*	blood brain barrier（BBB）（E）

欠陥状態	defect state（E）, Defektzustand（D）
血管性うつ病	vascular depression（E）
血管性頭痛	vascular headache（E）
血管性認知［痴呆］症	vascular dementia（E）
月経前緊張症候群	premenstrual tension syndrome（R. T. Frank）（E）
結実因子	precipitating factor（E）
欠神	absence（F）
結節性硬化症	tuberous sclerosis（E）
血統妄想	descent delusion（E）, Abstammungswahn（D）
ゲルストマン症候群	Gerstmann syndrome（E）
幻覚	hallucination（E）（F）, Halluzination（D）
幻覚剤	hallucinogen（E）
── 依存	hallucinogen dependence（E）
── 関連障害	hallucinogen-related disorders（DSM-IV）（E）
── 持続性知覚障害	hallucinogen persisting perception disorder（flashbacks）（E）
── 使用障害	hallucinogen use disorders（E）
── 中毒	hallucinogen intoxication（E）
── 中毒せん妄	hallucinogen intoxication delirium
── 誘発性気分障害	hallucinogen-induced mood disorders（E）
── 誘発性障害	hallucinogen-induced disorders（E）
── 誘発性精神病性障害	hallucinogen-induced psychotic disorders（E）
── 誘発性不安障害	hallucinogen-induced anxiety disorders（E）
── 乱用	hallucinogen abuse（E）
幻覚症	Halluzinose（C. Wernicke）（D）
幻覚発作	hallucinatory seizure（E）
衒奇（症）→わざとらしさ	
幻嗅	Geruchshalluzination（D）

幻嗅発作	olfactory hallucinatory seizure（E）
元型	Archetypus（C. G. Jung）（D）
原光景	primary scene（E），Urszene（D），scène originaire（F）
言語化	verbalization（E）
言語間代，語間代	logoclonia（E），Logoklonie（D）
言語緩慢*→発語緩慢*	
言語幻聴	verbal hallucination（E）
言語錯乱	Sprachverwirrtheit（D）
言語自動症	verbal automatism（E）
言語常同	Sprachstereotypie（D）
言語新作，造語（症）	neologism（E），Wortneubildung（D）
言語性精神運動幻覚	hallucination psychomotrice verbale（J. Séglas）（F）
言語中枢	speech center（E）
言語不当配列	acataphasia（E）
顕在記憶，外示記憶	explicit memory（E）
現在症診察表	present state examination（PSE）（E）
幻視	visual hallucination（E），Gesichtshalluzination（D）
幻（影）肢	phantom limb（E），Phantomglied（D）
顕示型精神病質者	Geltungsbedürftige（Psychopathen）（K. Schneider）（D）
原始感覚	protopathic sensation（E）
現実意識	Realitätsbewußtsein（D）
現実界	le réel（J. Lacan）（F）
現実感消失，離現実感	Derealisation（W. Mayer-Gross）（D）
現実機能	fonction du réel（P. Janet）（F）
現実原則［原理］	reality principle（E），Realitätsprinzip（D）
現実検討	reality testing（E），Realitätsprüfung（D）
現実見当識	reality orientation（E）
現実神経症	Aktualneurose（S. Freud）（D）

現実との生きた接触	contact vital avec la réalité（E. Minkowski）（F）
現実不安	Realangst（S. Freud）（D）
原始的防衛機制	primitive defence mechanism（E）
原始的理想化	primitive idealization（E）
原始反応	primitive reaction（E）
嫌酒薬，抗酒薬	antialcoholic agent（E）
現象学	phenomenology（E），Phäneomenologie（D），phénoménologie（F）
現象学的精神病理学	phänomenologische Psychopathologie（D）
顕示欲	Geltungsbedürfnis（D）
幻触	haptic hallucination，tactile hallucination（E），Berührungshalluzination（D）
幻声	Stimmenhören（D）
現存在分析	Daseinsanalyse（D）
幻聴	auditory hallucination（E），Gehörshalluzination（D）
幻聴発作	auditory hallucinatory seizure（E）
限定帰責能力	verminderte Zurechnungsfähigkeit（D）
限定責任能力	verminderte Schuldfähigkeit（D）
減動*→運動減少（症）*	
見当識	orientation（E），Orientierung（D）
原発性精神錯乱	confusion mentale primitive（P. Chaslin）（F）
原発てんかん	primary epilepsy（E）
原不安	Urangst（S. Freud）（D）
健忘	amnesia（E）
健忘失語	amnes(t)ic aphasia（E）
健忘症候群	amnes(t)ic syndrome（E）
幻味	Geschmackshalluzination（D），gustatory hallucination（E）
権利擁護	advocacy（E）

こ

語唖	word dumbness（E）
口愛（性）	orality（E）
口愛期	oral phase（E）
口愛性格	oral character（E）
行為および情緒の混合性障害→素行および情動の混合性障害	
行為障害→素行障害	
行為心迫	Tatendrang（D）
行為能力	Geschäftsfähigkeit, Handlungsfähigkeit（D）, contractual capacity（E）
行為抑制	conduct retardation（E）, Hemmung（D）
抗うつ薬	antidepressant（E）
光音症	Lichtphonismus（D）
構音障害*	dysarthria（E）, Artikulationsstörung（D）
構音不能	anarthria（E）, anarthrie（F）
鉤回発作	uncinate fits（H. Jackson）（E）
口蓋ミオクローヌス	palatal myoclonus（E）
高感情表出家族	family with high expressed emotion（EE）（E）
交感性失行	sympathetic apraxia（E）
高危険児法	high risk study（E）
後弓反張→弓なり緊張	
拘禁昏迷	Haftstupor（D）
拘禁精神病	prison psychosis（E）, Haftpsychose（D）
拘禁反応	prison reaction（E）, Haftreaktion（D）
拘禁保護，収容保護	custodial care（E）
後屈小発作	Retropulsiv-petit-mal（D. Janz）（D）
抗けいれん薬	anticonvulsant（E）
攻撃（性）	aggression（E）
光原てんかん	photogenic epilepsy（E）
後見人	guardian（E）

恍惚	ecstasy（E）
抗コリン薬	anticholinergic drug（E）
交際恐怖	homilophobia（E）
抗酒薬→嫌酒薬	
甲状腺精神病	thyreogenic psychosis（E）
高照度光療法	bright light treatment，phototherapy（E）
高所恐怖	acrophobia（E）
構成失行	constructive apraxia（E），constructional apraxia（E），konstruktive Apraxie（D）
構成失書	constructional agraphia，constructive agraphia（E）
抗精神病薬	antipsychotic drug（E），antipsychotics（E）
向精神薬	psychotropic drug（E）
構成（的）面接法	structural interview（E）
考想可視，思考可視	Gedankensichtbarwerden（Halbey，K）（D），visible thoughts（E）
考想化声，思考化声	Gedankenlautwerden（Störring，G）（D），audible thoughts（E）
構造化面接	structured interview（E）
考想察知，思考察知	Gedankenverstandenwerden（D），mind reading（E）
考想吹入，思考吹入	Gedankeneningebung（D），thought insertion（E）
考想奪取，思考奪取	Gedankenentzug（D），thought withdrawal（E）
考想伝播，思考伝播	Gedankenausbreitung（D），thought broadcasting（E）
考想反響，思考反響	Gedankenecho（D），thought echo（E），écho de la pensée（F）
考想貧困，思考貧困	Gedankenarmut（D）
構造分析	Strukturanalyse（K. Birnbaum）（D）
好訴者	Querulant（D）

好訴妄想	querulous delusion（E）, Querulantenwahn（D）
交代意識	alternating consciousness（E）, alternierendes Bewußtsein（D）
交代狂気（歴史用語）	folie alterne（F）
交替勤務睡眠障害	sleep disturbance of shift worker（E）
交代人格	alternating personality（E）, alternierende Persönlichkeit（D）
抗てんかん薬	antiepileptics（E）, antiepileptic drug（E）
行動	behavior（E）, Verhalten（D）, comportement（F）
行動化	acting out（E）
行動療法	behavior therapy（E）
抗認知［痴呆］症薬, 向知性薬	nootropics（E）, nootropic drug（E）, cognitive enhancer（E）
孔脳症	porencephaly（E）
荒廃	deterioration（E）, Verbödung（D）
広汎性発達障害	pervasive developmental disorders（DSM-III）（E）
向反発作	adversive seizure（E）
抗不安薬	antianxiety drug, anxiolytic drug（E）, anxiolytics（E）
口部顔面失行	buccofacial apraxia（E）
口部傾向→口運び傾向	
項部硬直	nuchal stiffness（E）, Nackenstarre（D）
口部ジスキネジー［ジスキネジア］*	oral dyskinesia（E）
口部小発作	Oral-Petit mal（D. Janz）（D）
後方失語	posterior aphasia（E）
肛門愛	anality（E）
肛門愛期	anal phase［stage］（E）
肛門期性格	anal character（E）
肛門性交	sodomy（E）
合理化	rationalization（E）

合理的了解	rationales Verstehen（D）
交流分析	transactional analysis（E. Berne）（E）
コカイン	cocaine（E）
——依存	cocaine dependence（E）
——関連障害	cocaine-related disorders（DSM-IV）（E）
——（依存）症	cocainism（E）
——使用障害	cocaine use disorders（E）
——中毒	cocaine intoxication（E）
——中毒せん妄	cocaine intoxication delirium（E）
——誘発性気分障害	cocaine-induced mood disorder（E）
——誘発性障害	cocaine-induced disorders（E）
——誘発性睡眠障害	cocaine-sleep disorder（E）
——誘発性性機能不全	cocaine-induced sexual dysfunction（E）
——誘発性精神病性障害	cocaine-induced psychotic disorder（E）
——誘発性不安障害	cocaine-induced anxiety disorder（E）
——乱用	cocaine abuse（E）
——離脱	cocaine withdrawal（E）
語間代→言語間代	
誤記憶	allomnesia（E）
語義失語（井村恒郎）	semantic aphasia（E）
呼吸関連睡眠障害	breathing-related sleep disorder（E）
国際疾病分類（世界保健機構）	International Classification of Diseases（ICD）（WHO）（E）
語健忘	word amnesia, word finding disturbance（E）
心構えの障害	Einstellungsstörung（D）
心の理論	theory of mind（E）
ゴーシェ病	Gaucher disease（E）
固執傾向	Beharrungsneigung（D）
固縮*，硬直*，強剛*，強直*	rigidity, stiffness（E）
語唱	verbigeration（E）
個人精神療法	individual psychotherapy（E）

こ

コース立方体組み合わせテスト	Kohs blocks test（E）
語性錯語	verbal paraphasia（E）
コタール症候群	syndrome de Cotard（J. Cotard）（F），Cotard syndrome（E）
誇大妄想	grandiose delusion，megalomania（E），expansiver Wahn，Größenwahn（D），délire de grandeur（F），mégalomanie（F）
固着	fixation（E），Fixierung（D）
固着観念	fixed idea（E）
骨相学	phrenology（E）
言葉のサラダ	word salad（E），Wortsalat（D）
言葉もれ，語漏	logorrh(o)ea（E）
コーネル・メディカル・インデックス	Cornell Medical Index（CMI）（E）
こびと幻覚	lilliputian hallucination（E）
コーピング，対処	coping（E）
コミュニケーション障害	communication disorder（E）
コメディカル	co-medical（E）
語盲	word blindness（E）
コモビディティ　共存（症），併存（症）	comorbidity（E）
コリンエステラーゼ阻害薬	cholinesterase inhibitor（E）
コルサコフ症候群	Korsakoff syndrome（E）
コルサコフ精神病	Korsakoff psychosis（E）
コルネリア・デ・ランゲ症候群	Cornelia de Lange syndrome（E）
コロ	koro（E）
語呂あわせ	Wortspielerei（D）
語聾	word deafness（E）
混合状態	Mischzustand（W. Weygandt）（D），mixed state（E）
混合精神病	mixed psychosis（E），Mischpsychose（D）
混合性超皮質性失語（症）	mixed transcortical aphasia（E）
混合性特異的発達障害	mixed specific developmental disorder（E）

混合性不安抑うつ障害	mixed anxiety and depressive disorder（E）
コンサルテーション・リエゾン精神医学	consultation-liaison psychiatry（E）
昏睡	coma（E），Koma（D）
コンパートメント・モデル	compartment model（E）
コンピューター断層撮影	computed tomography, computerized tomography（CT）（E）
コンプライアンス，服薬遵守	compliance（E，F）
コンプレックス，（心的）複合（体）	Komplex（D），complex（E）
昏迷	stupor（E），Stupor（D）
昏蒙	benumbness（E），Benommenheit（D）
困惑	bewilderment，perplexity（E），Ratlosigkeit（D）

さ

災害神経症	accident neurosis（E），Unfallneurose（D）
催奇性	tetratogenicity（E）
細菌恐怖	bacillophobia（E）
罪業妄想，罪責妄想	delusion of guilt（E），Sündenwahn，Versündigungswahn（D）
サイコオンコロジー，精神腫瘍学	psychooncology（E）
サイコドラマ，心理劇	psychodrama（E）
サイコネフロロジー	psychonephrology（E）
最重度精神遅滞	profound mental retardation（E）
再生，想起	reproduction（E），Reproduktion（D）
罪責感	guilt feeling（E），Schuldgefühl（D）
最早発痴呆（歴史用語）	dementia praecocissima（De Sanctis）（L）
在宅ケア	home care（E）
再認	recognition（E），Wiedererkennung（D）
再燃	relapse（E）
再発	recurrence（E），Rezidiv（D）
催眠	hypnosis（E）

催眠後暗示	post-hypnotic suggestion（E）
催眠分析	hypnoanalysis（E）
催眠療法	hypnotherapy（E）
サーカディアンリズム→概日リズム	
作業心迫	Beschäftigungsdrang（D）
作業せん妄，職業せん妄	occupational delirium（E），Beschäftigungsdelirium（D）
作業療法	occupational therapy（E），Arbeitstherapie，Beschäftigungstherapie（D），ergothérapie（F）
作業療法士	occupational therapist（OT）（E）
錯感覚*	paresthesia（E）
錯語	paraphasia（E）
錯行（為）	parapraxia（E），Fehlleistung（D）
錯書	paragraphia（E）
錯触	Berührungsillusion（D）
錯読	paralexia（E）
錯文法	paragrammatism（E）
錯味	Geschmacksillusion（D）
錯眠→パラソムニア	
錯乱	confusion（E），Verwirrtheit（D）
錯乱精神病	Verwirrtheitspsychose（D）
錯乱躁病	verworrene Manie（D）
錯論理	paralogia（E）
作話	confabulation（E），Konfabulation，Fabulieren（D）
させられ現象，作為現象	gemachtes Phänomen（D）
させられ体験，作為体験	gemachtes Erlebnis（D）
サチリアージス	satyriasis（E）
錯覚	illusion（E）
サディズム→加虐性愛	
作動［働］記憶，ワーキングメモリー	working memory（E）
作動薬，作動物質→アゴニスト	
里親保護［ケア］	foster home care（E）

悟り体験	Erleuchtungserlebnis（D）
詐病	malingering（E），simulation（E），Simulation（D）
左右障害	right-left disorientation（E），Rechtslinksstörung（D）
残遺（型）統合失調症	residual schizophrenia（E）
残遺てんかん	residual epilepsy（E）
残遺妄想	Residualwahn（D）
三環系抗うつ薬	tricyclic antidepressant，tricyclics（E）
産業精神保健	occupational mental health（E）
残語	rest word（E），Wortrest（D）
産後うつ病	postpartum depression（E）
産褥うつ病	puerperal depression（E）
産褥期精神障害	puerperal mental disorders（E）
産褥精神病	puerperal psychosis（E），Wochenbettpsychose（D）
算数障害	mathematics disorder（DSM-IV），arithmetic disorder（ICD-10）（E）
三相波	triphasic waves（E）

し

視運動性眼振*	optokinetic nystagmus（OKN）（E）
自我	ego（E），Ich（D），moi（F）
自我意識	Ichbewußtsein（D）
自我異質性	ego-dystonic（E）
自我感情	Ichgefühl（D）
自我境界	ego boundary（E），Ichgrenzen（P. Federn）（D）
視覚運動失調	visuomotor ataxia（E）
視覚失調	optic ataxia（E），optische Ataxie（M. Balint）（D）
視覚失認	visual agnosia（E）
視覚性失見当（識）	visual disorientation（E）
視覚性注意障害	disturbance of visual attention（E）
視覚発作	visual seizure（E）

視覚誘発電位	visual evoked potential（VEP）（E）
自我収縮	Ich-Anachorese（W. Th. Winkler）（D）
自我障害	Ichstörung（D）
自我親和性	ego-syntonic（E）
自我性	Ichhaftigkeit（D）
自我体験	Icherlebnis（D）
自我同一性	ego identity（E. H. Erikson）（E）
自我本能	instinct of self-preservation（E）
しかめ顔	grimace, grimas（E）, Grimassieren, Grimasse（D）
自我理想	ego ideal（E）
自我漏洩（性）症状	egorrh(o)ea symptoms（藤縄昭）（E）
時間意識	Zeitbewußtsein（D）
時間緩慢現象	Zeitlupenphänomen（D）
時間失見当	temporal disorientation（E）, zeitliche Desorientiertheit（D）
時間迅速現象	Zeitrafferphänomen（D）
時間制限精神療法	time-limited psychotherapy（E）
時間精神医学	chronopsychiatry（E）
時間生物学	chronobiology（E）
弛緩性麻痺*	flaccid paralysis（E）
弛緩（性）メランコリー	melancholia attonita（L）
時間体験	Zeiterleben（D）
時間療法	chronotherapy（E）
識覚	sensorium（E）
磁気共鳴画像	magnetic resonance imaging（MRI）（E）
磁気共鳴血管造影（法）	magnetic resonance angiography（MRA）（E）
磁気共鳴スペクトル法	magnetic resonance spectroscopy（MRS）（E）
色彩失認	Farbenagnosie（D）
色情症，恋愛妄想	erotomania（E）, érotomanie（F）
色聴	color-hearing（E）, Farbenhören（D）
児戯的	läppisch（D）

色名［彩］呼称障害［不能］，色名［彩］失名辞	color anomia（E）
嗜銀顆粒性認知［痴呆］症	argy[i]rophilic grain dementia（AGD）（E）
視空間失認	visual-spatial agnosia（E）
軸性健忘	axial amnesia（E）
刺激性	irritability（E），Reizbarkeit（D）
刺激性衰弱	irritable weakness（E），reizbare Schwäche（D）
自己愛，ナルシ（シ）ズム	narcissism（E）
自己愛（性）パーソナリティ［人格］障害	narcissistic personality disorder（DSM-III）（E）
自己暗示	autosuggestion（E）
自己意識	Selbstbewußtsein（D），self consciousness（E）
思考可視→考想可視	
思考化声→考想化声	
思考干渉	Gedankenbeeinflußung（D）
思考察知→考想察知	
思考散乱	Inkohärenz（D）
思考障害	thought disorder，disturbance of thought（E），Denkstörung（D）
思考吹入→考想吹入	
持効性抗精神病薬	sustained release dosage form of antipsychotics（E）
思考制止，思考抑制	inhibition of thought（E），Denkhemmung（D）
思考促迫	Gedankendrängen（D）
思考怠惰，考え不精	Denkfaulheit（D），laziness of thinking（E）
思考奪取→考想奪取	
思考伝播→考想伝播	
思考途絶	blocking of thought（E），Denksperrung（D）
思考飛躍	Gedankensprung（D）

思考貧困→考想貧困	
思考滅裂，滅裂思考	incoherence of thought（E）, Zerfahrenheit（D）
自己関係づけ	reference upon one's own self（E）, Eigenbeziehung（D）
事故傾性	accident proneness（E）
自己志向性	self-directed（E）
自己視（症）→自己像幻視	
自己視線恐怖	fear of eye-to-eye confrontation（E）
自己臭恐怖	fear of emitting body odor（E）
自己所属感	sentiment d'appropriation au moi（F）
自己所属性	Meinhaftigkeit（D）
自己所属剥奪感	dépossession（F）
自己身体部位失認	autotopagnosia（E）
自己像幻視	autoscopy（E）, Autoskopie, Heautoskopie（D）, héautoscopie（F）
自己疎隔感	Entfremdungsgefühl（D）
自己中心性	self-centered（E）
自己同一性→自我同一性	
自己描写	Selbstschilderung（D）
自己保存欲	Selbsterhaltungstrieb（D）
時差症候群	jet lag syndrome（E）
自殺	suicide（E）, Selbstmord, Suizid（D）
自殺企図	attempt of suicide（E）, Selbstmordversuch（D）
自殺念慮，希死念慮	idea of suicide（E）, Selbstmordgedanke（D）
支持	support（E）
指示試験*	past-pointing test（E）
支持的精神療法	supportive psychotherapy（E）
四肢麻痺*	tetraplegia（E）
思春期危機	Pubertätskrise（D）
思春期妄想症	adolescent paranoia（E）, Pubertätsparanoia（D）
思春期やせ症	Pubertätsmagersucht（D）

自傷	self-mutilation（E），Selbstverletzung，Selbstverstümmelung（D）
事象関連電位	event-related potential（E）
視床認知［痴呆］症	thalamic dementia（E）
自助グループ，セルフヘルプグループ	self-help group（E）
自信欠乏型（精神病質者）	Selbstunsichere（Psychopathen）（K. Schneider）（D）
ジスキネジー，ジスキネジア*	dyskinesia（E）
ジストニー，ジストニア*	dystonia（E）
字性錯語	literal paraphasia（E）
自生思考	autochthonous idea（E），autochthones Denken（D）
姿勢時振戦*	postural tremor（E）
姿勢反射*	postural reflex（E）
姿勢保持困難*	asterixis（E）
姿勢発作	postural seizure（E）
姿勢めまい	postural vertigo（E）
自責	self-accusation（E），Selbstvorwurf（D）
肢節運動失行	limb-kinetic apraxia（E）
施設化	institutionalization（E）
施設症	institutionalism，hospitalism（E）
施設神経症	institutional neurosis（E）
施設内リハビリテーション	institutional rehabilitation（E）
自然な自明性	natürliche Selbstverständlichkeit（W. Blankenburg）（D）
持続睡眠	Dauerschlaf（D）
持続性不眠	persistent insomnia（E）
持続性妄想性障害	persistent delusional disorders（E）
持続浴	Dauerbad（D）
自体愛	autoerotism（E）
死体性愛，屍姦	necrophilia（E）
死態反射	Totstellreflex（D）
舌語り	glossolalia（E），Zungenreden（D）
私宅監置	confinement at one's family home（E）

失音楽	amusia（E）
失音調	dysprosody（E）
失外套症候群	apallisches Syndrom（E. Kretschmer）（D），apallic syndrome（E）
疾患	disease（E）
疾患隠蔽	dissimulation（E）
失感情（言語）症，アレキシシミア，アレキシサイミア	alexithymia（E），Alexithymie（D）
疾患単位	Krankheitseinheit（D），disease entity（E）
疾患の負荷	Leidensdruck（D）
実験神経症	experimental neurosis（E）
実験精神病	experimental psychosis（E）
失見当（識）	disorientation（E），Desorientiertheit（D）
失語（症）	aphasia（E），Aphasie（D）
失行（症）	apraxia（E），Apraxie（D）
失構音，構音不能，アナルトリー	anarthria（E）
失行失認	apractognosia（E）
失語（症）検査	test of aphasia（E）
失算	acalculia（E）
失書	agraphia（E）
失象徴	asymbolia（E）
失神	syncope（E），Ohnmacht（D）
失声（症）	aphonia（E），Aphonie（D）
実存うつ病	existentielle Depression（H. Häfner）（D）
実存分析	Existenzanalyse（D）
実体（的）意識性	leibhaftige Bewußtheit（D）
実体性	Leibhaftigkeit（D）
失調性歩行*	ataxic gait（E）
失読	alexia（E）
嫉妬妄想	delusion of jealousy（E），Eifersuchtswahn（D）
失認	agnosia（E）

失文法	agrammatism（E）
疾病恐怖	nosophobia, pathophobia（E）
疾病（性）	illness（E）
疾病否認	denial of illness（E）, Verneinung der Krankheit（D）
疾病分類学	nosology（E）
疾病への逃避	flight into illness（E）, Flucht in die Krankheit（D）
疾病無関心	anosodiaphoria（E）
疾病利得	Krankheitsgewinn（D）, gain from illness（E）
失歩	abasia（E）
失名辞（詞）失語（症）	anomic aphasia（E）
質問紙法	questionnaire method（E）
質問癖	Fragesucht（D）
失立	astasia（E）
失立発作	astatic seizure（E）
指定病院	designated hospital（E）
シデナム舞踏病*	Sydenham chorea（E）
自伝記憶	autobiographic memory（E）
児童（期）神経症	childhood neurosis（E）, Kinderneurose（D）
児童（期）（小児）統合失調症	childhood schizophrenia（E）, Kinderschizophrenie（D）
児童虐待	child abuse（E）
自動思考	automatic thought（E）
自動症	automatism（E）
自動書記	automatic writing（E）
児童精神医学	child psychiatry（E）, Kinderpsychiatrie（D）
児童相談所	child guidance center（E）
児童福祉法	Child Welfare Law（E）
シナプス	synapse（E）
シヌクレイノパチー	synucleinopathy（E）

支配観念，優格観念	dominierende Vorstellung，überwertige Idee（D），overvalue idea（E）
自発語	Spontansprechen（D）
自発性欠乏	Spontaneitätsmangel（D）
自発性消失	aspontaneity，loss of initiative（E），Initiativelosigkeit（D）
自発入院	voluntary admission（E）
四半（分）盲*	quadrantanopsia（E）
自閉（症）	autism（E），Autismus（D）
自閉性障害	autistic disorder（E）
自閉的精神病質	autistische Psychopathie（H. Asperger）（D）
嗜癖	addiction（E），Sucht（D）
死別反応	bereavement（E）
司法精神医学	forensic psychiatry（E），gerichtliche Psychiatrie（D），psychiatrie medico-légale（F）
嗜眠	lethargy（E），Schlafsucht（D）
シャイ-ドレーガー症候群*	Shy-Drager syndrome（E）
社会因性	sociogenic（E）
社会化	socialization（E）
社会（的）寛解	soziale Remission（D），social remission（E）
社会記憶	mémoire sociale（J. Delay）（F）
社会生活技能訓練（法）	social skills training（SST）（E）
社会精神医学	social psychiatry（E）
社会測定法	sociometry（J. L. Moreno）（E）
社会的再適応評定スケール	social readjustment rating scale（E）
社会的・職業的機能評価尺度	social and occupational functioning assessment scale（E）
社会的入院	admission with social reasons（E）
社会的入院患者	inpatients with social reasons（E）
社会的不利，ハンディキャップ	handicap（E）
社会脳	social brain（E）
社会病理学	social pathology（E）

社会福祉	social welfare（E）
社会復帰→リハビリテーション	
社会復帰準備期（森田療法）	daily living training stage（Morita therapy）（E）
ジャクソン学説	Jacksonism（E）
ジャクソン型発作	Jacksonian seizure（E）
ジャクソンマーチ	Jacksonian march（E）
灼熱痛	causalgia（E）
若年欠神てんかん	juvenile absence epilepsy（E）
若年進行麻痺	juvenile paresis（E）
若年性アルツハイマー病	juvenile Alzheimer disease（E）
若年ミオクロニーてんかん	juvenile myoclonic epilepsy（E）
社交恐怖	social phobia（DSM-III）（E）
社交不安障害	social anxiety disorder（DSM-IV）（E）
シャーマニズム	shamanism（E）
赦免妄想	Begnadigungswahn（D），delusion of amnesty（E）
ジャルゴン失語	jargon aphasia（E）
シャルル ボネ症候群	Charles Bonnet syndrome（E）
獣化妄想	Tierverwandlungswahn（D），zoanthropy（E）
獣姦	Sodomie（D），bestiality（E）
周期嘔吐	cyclic vomiting（E）
周期気分変調	periodische Verstimmung（D）
周期傾眠症	periodic somnolence（E）
周期嗜眠症	periodische Schlafsucht（D）
周期性四肢運動障害	periodic limb movement disorder（E）
周期精神病	periodic psychosis（E）
周期性同期性放電	periodic synchronous discharge（PSD）（E）
宗教妄想	religious delusion（E）
醜形恐怖	dysmorphophobia（E）
重作業期（森田療法）	heavy work stage（Morita therapy）（E）
収集症	collectomania（E），Sammelsucht（D）
収集癖	collectionism（E），collectionnisme（F）

修正型電気けいれん［通電］療法	modified electroconvulsive therapy (m-ECT)（E）
集団精神療法	group psychotherapy（E）
集団ヒステリー	Massenhysterie（D），mass hysteria（E）
縦断法	longitudinal study（E）
執着気質	Immodithymie（Immobilithymie）（下田光造）（D）
集中治療室精神病	intensive care unit psychosis, ICU psychosis（E）
重度精神遅滞	severe mental retardation（E）
重複記憶錯誤	reduplicative paramnesia（E），reduplizierende Paramnesie（A. Pick）（D）
修復作用→償い	
終末睡眠	terminal sleep（E）
週末病院	weekend hospital（E）
就眠儀式	Schlafzeremonie（D）
就眠困難→入眠困難	
収容保護→拘禁保護	
自由連想（法）	free association（E）
受刑能力	Straffähigkeit（D）
守護妄想	délire de protection（F）
授産施設	sheltered work institution for mentally handicapped person（E）
主軸症状→中軸症状	
手指失認	finger agnosia（E）
呪術思考	magical thinking（E）
手掌おとがい反射*	palmomental reflex（E）
主訴	chief complaint（E），Hauptklage（D）
術後精神病	postoperative psychosis（E）
出産（心的）外傷	birth trauma（E）
出典健忘	source amnesia（E）
出眠幻覚	hypnopompic hallucination（E）

受動-攻撃（性）パーソナリティ［人格］障害	passive-aggressive personality disorder（DSM-III）（E）
授乳期精神病	Laktationspsychose（D）
守秘義務	confidentiality（E）
シューブ	Schub（D）
樹木画テスト→バウムテスト	
受容	acceptance（E）
受容失語	receptive aphasia（E）
受容性言語障害	receptive language disorder（ICD-10）（E）
受容体，レセプター	receptor（E）
受容-表出混合性言語障害	mixed receptive-expressive language disorder（DSM-IV）（E）
循環気質，気分循環症	cyclothymia（ICD-10）（E）
循環狂気（歴史用語）	folie circulaire（J-P. Falret）（F）
循環精神病（歴史用語）	zirkuläre Psychose（D）
循環性統合失調症	cyclic schizopherenia（E）
循環病（症）	Zyklothymie（D）
循環病質	cycloid（E）
準禁治産→被保佐	
純粋欠陥	reiner Defekt（G. Huber）（D）
純粋健忘	pure amnesia（E）
純粋語啞	pure word-dumbness（E）
純粋語聾	pure word-deafness（E）
純粋失書	pure agraphia（E）
純粋失読	pure alexia, alexia without agraphia（E）
純粋小発作	pure petit mal（E）
昇華	sublimation（E）
浄化→カタルシス	
障害者自立支援法	services and supports for persons with disabilities act（E）
上機嫌症→多幸症	
状況因，発病状況論	Situagenie（D）

状況関連性発作，機会発作	situation-related seizure, occasional seizures（E）, Gelegenheitsanfälle（D）
状況失見当	situative Desorientierung（D）
衝撃小発作	Impulsiv-petit-mal（D. Janz）（D）
条件づけ	conditioning（E）
条件反射	conditioned reflex（E）
症候性	symptomatic（E）
症候性てんかん	symptomatic epilepsy（E）
症候性統合失調症	symptomatic schizophrenia（E）
小視症	micropsia（E）
小字症	micrographia（E）
使用失認	agnosie d'utilisation（J. Morlaas）（F）
常習犯罪者	habitual criminal（E）
症状精神病	symptomatic psychosis（E）
症状転嫁	transitivism（E）
症状評価尺度→精神症状評価尺度	
情性欠如型（精神病質者）	Gemütlose（Psychopathen）（K. Schneider）（D）
小精神療法	brief psychotherapy（E）, kleine Psychotherapie（D）
情操	sentiment（E）, höheres Gefühl（D）
冗長	Weitschweifigkeit（D）
象徴化	symbolization（E）
焦点運動発作	focal motor seizure（E）
焦点症状	focal symptom（E）
焦点発作	focal seizure（E）
情動	affect, emotion（E）, Affekt, Emotion（D）, affect, émotion（F）
常同運動障害，常同症／性癖障害	stereotype movement disorder, stereotype/habit disorder（E）
衝動行為	impulsive act（E）, impulsive Handlung（D）
情動昏迷	Affektstupor, Emotionsstupor（D）
常同姿勢	Haltungsstereotypie（D）

情動失禁	emotional incontinence (E), Affektinkontinenz (D)
小頭症	microcephaly(ia) (E)
常同症	stereotypy (E)
情動性	Affektivität (D)
衝動制御の障害	impulse-control disorder (E)
情動性緊張消失	Affekttonusverlust (D)
情動不安定	Affektlabilität (D)
情動不安定パーソナリティ［人格］障害	emotionally unstable personality disorder (E)
情動麻痺	Emotionslähmung (D)
情動抑うつ	emotionale Depression (K. Schneider) (D)
小児［児童］うつ病	childhood depression (E)
小児期崩壊性障害	childhood disintegrative disorder (DSM-IV) (E)
小児欠神てんかん	childhood absence epilepsy (E)
小児症	infantilism (E)
小児性愛	pedophilia (E)
小児の過剰不安障害	overanxious disorder of child (E)
小児への性的虐待	sexual abuse of child (E)
小児への無視	neglect of child (E)
小児または青年の反社会的行動	child and adolescent antisocial behavior (E)
小脳回（症）	microgyria (E)
小舞踏病	chorea minor (E)
小発作	petit mal (F)
小発作（波）異型	petit mal variant (F. A. & E. L. Gibbs) (E)
小発作異型欠神	petit mal variant absence (E)
小発作欠神	petit mal absence (E)
小発作重積状態	petit mal status (E)
消耗うつ病［抑うつ］	Erschöpfungsdepression (P. Kielholz) (D)
消耗神経症	Erschöpfungsneurose (D)

除外診断	diagnosis by exclusion（E）
初期叫声	initial cry（E），Initialschrei（D）
職親	vocational parent（E）
職親（委託）制度（解説用語）	foster employer system（臺弘），aid system for employer（岡上和雄），labor resettlement system（E）
職業上の問題	occupational problem（E）
職業せん妄→作業せん妄	
食事恐怖	sitiophobia（E）
植物状態	vegetative state（E）
植物神経症	vegetative Neurose（D）
食糞	coprophagia（E）
触法精神障害者	mentally handicapped person who engages illegal conduct and comes under the protection of the law（E）
食欲異常	dysorexia（E）
食欲過剰	hyperorexia（E）
書痙	writer's cramp, writer's spasm（E），Schreibkrampf（D）
書字障害	dysgraphia（E）
書字反復	paligraphia（E）
書字表出障害	disorder of written expression（E）
女性オルガズム障害	female orgasmic disorder（E）
女性化	feminization（E），effeminatio（L）
女性恐怖	gyn(a)ephobia（E）
女性色情症	nymphomania（E）
触覚失語	tactile aphasia（E）
触覚失認	tactile agnosia（E）
触覚消去	tactile extinction（E）
除脳姿勢*	decerebrate posture（E）
徐波	slow wave（E）
徐波群発	slow burst（E）
除皮質姿勢*	decorticate posture（E）
除覆法	aufdeckende Methode（D）
初老期認知［痴呆］症	presenile dementia（E）

自律訓練（法）	autogenes Training（J. H. Schultz）（D），autogenic training（E）
自律神経失調症	autonomic dystonia（E）
自律神経発作	autonomic seizure（E）
支離滅裂	incoherence（E），Zerfahrenheit（D），Inkohärenz（D）
シルダー病*（歴史用語）	Schilder disease（E）
ジル・ドゥ・ラ・トゥレット症候群→トゥレット症候群	
事例性	caseness（E）
思路	Gedankengang（D）
思路障害	Gedankengangstörung（D）
心因うつ病，心因抑うつ	psychogenic depression（E）
心因症	Psychogenie（R. Sommer）（D）
心因性	psychogenic（E）
心因性嘔吐（症）	psychogenic vomiting（E）
心因性加重	psychogenic overlay（E），psychogene Überlagerung（D）
心因性健忘	psychogenic amnesia（E）
心因性昏迷	psychogenic stupor（E）
心因性精神病	psychogenic psychosis（E）
心因性多飲（症）	psychogenic polydipsia（E）
心因性遁走	psychogenic fugue（E）
心因反応	psychogenic reaction（E）
進化	evolution（H. Jackson）（E）
侵害妄想	delusion of injury（E），Beeinträchtigungwahn（D），délire de préjudice（F）
人格異常，異常人格	abnorme Persönlichkeit（D），personnalité pathologique（F）
人格障害，パーソナリティ障害	personality disorder（ICD-9, DSM-III）（E）
人格水準低下	Persönlichkeitsniveausenkung（D）
人格の尖鋭化	Zuspitzung der Persönlichkeit（D）

人格発展の屈折	Knick der Persönlichkeitsentwicklung（D）
人格反応	Persönlichkeitsreaktion（D）
人格変化	personality change（E），Persönlichkeitsveränderung，Wesens(ver)änderung（D）
人格崩壊	Persönlichkeitszerfall（D）
新規健忘，エクムネジー	ecmnesia（E），ecmnésie（F）
心気症	hypochondriasis（E），Hypochondrie（D）
心気妄想	hypochondriacal delusion（E），hypochondrischer Wahn（D）
神経因性膀胱	neurogenic bladder（E）
神経科学	neuroscience（E）
神経（病）学	neurology（E）
神経原線維変化型老年認知［痴呆］症	senile dementia with neurofibrillary tangle（SD-NFT）（E）
神経弛緩薬	neuroleptica（L）
神経質	Nervosität（M. Morita）（D），Shinkeishitsu（森田正馬）（J）
神経遮断薬	neuroplegica（L），neuroleptics（E）
神経遮断薬悪性症候群	neuroleptic malignant syndrome（E）
神経遮断薬誘発性急性アカシジア	neuroleptic-induced akathisia（E）
神経遮断薬誘発性急性ジストニー	neuroleptic-induced acute dystonia（E）
神経遮断薬誘発性遅発性ジスキネジー	neuroleptic-induced tardive dyskinesia（E）
神経遮断薬誘発性パーキンソニズム	neuroleptic-induced parkinsonism（E）
神経症	neurosis（E），Neurose（D），névrose（F）
神経症性うつ病，神経症性抑うつ	neurotic depression（E），neurotische Depression（D）
神経症的加重	neurotic overlay（E）
神経症的習癖	neurotic habituation（E）
神経心理学	neuropsychology（E）
神経心理学的検査	neuropsychological examination（E）

神経衰弱	neurasthenia (E)
神経精神医学	neuropsychiatry (E)
神経性大［過］食症	bulimia nervosa (L)
神経性無食欲症，神経性食欲不振症	anorexia nervosa (L)
神経伝達物質	neurotransmitter (E)
神経毒	neurotoxin (E)
神経梅毒	neurosyphillis (E), Neurosyphillis (D)
神経発達障害仮説	neurodevelopmental hypothesis (E)
神経病理学	neuropathology (E)
神経ベーチェット症候群（病）*	neuro-Behçet syndrome (disease) (E)
神経ペプチド	neuropeptide (E)
神経薬理学	neuropsychopharmacology (E)
唇語	Lippensprache (D)
進行性核上性麻痺*	progressive supranuclear palsy (PSP) (E)
進行性多巣性白質脳症*	progressive multifocal leukoencephalopathy (PML) (E)
進行麻痺	general paresis, general paralysis (E), progressive Paralyse (D)
紳士詐欺師	Hochstapler (D)
新ジャクソン学説	néo-Jacksonisme (F)
侵襲学	agressology (E), agressologie (F)
心身医学	psychosomatic medicine (E)
心神耗弱	diminished responsibility (E), verminderte Zurechnungsfähigkeit (D)
心身症	psychosomatic disease (E), psychosomatische Krankheit (D)
心身障害者対策基本法	Fundamental Law for Countermeasures Concerning Mentally and Physically Handicapped Persons (E)
心神消耗	weak minded (E)
心身相関	psychosomatic correlation (E)

心神喪失	noncompos mentis, irresponsibility（E）, Zurechnungsunfähigkeit（D）
心神喪失者医療観察法	Act on Medical Care and Treatment for Persons who have caused serious Cases under the Condition of Insanity（E）
真性幻覚	true hallucination（E）, echte Halluzination（D）
真性てんかん	genuine epilepsy（E）
真性統合失調症	Echteschizophrenie（D）
真性妄想	echter Wahn（D）
振戦	tremor（E）, Zittern（D）, tremblement（F）
振戦せん妄	delirium tremens（L）
振戦麻痺*（歴史用語）	paralysis agitans（L）
心臓神経症	cardiac neurosis（E）, Herzneurose（D）
深層心理学	depth psychology（E）, Tiefenpsychologie（D）, psychologie en profondeur（F）
身体意識	Somatopsyche（C. Wernicke）（D）
身体依存	physical dependence（E）
身体化	somatization（E）, Somatisierung（D）
身体化障害	somatization disorder（E）
身体管理精神医学	medical psychiatry（E）
身体自我	Körper-Ich（D）
身体失認	asomatognosia（E）
身体醜形障害	body dysmorphic disorders（E）
身体障害者福祉法	law for the welfare of the physically handicapped（E）
身体症状	somatic symptoms（E）
身体図式	body schema（E）, Körperschema（D）
身体像	body image（E）
身体的虐待, 肉体的虐待	physical abuse（E）

身体に基礎をおく精神病	körperlich begründbare Psychose（K. Schneider）（D）
身体認知障害	somatognostic disorder（E）
身体表現性障害	somatoform disorder（E）
身体療法	physical therapy（treatment）（E）
身体論者	Somatiker（D）
診断基準	diagnostic criteria（E）
心的エネルギー	psychic energy（E），énergie psychique（F）
心的外傷，トラウマ	psychic trauma（E）
心的外傷後ストレス障害	post-traumatic stress disorder（PTSD）（E）
心的決定論	psychic determinism（E）
心的反芻	rumination mentale（P. Janet）（F）
伸展性*	extensibilité（F）
伸展対麻痺*	paraplegia in extension（E）
心内失調	intrapsychische Ataxie（E. Stransky）（D）
心迫	impulsion（E），Drang（D）
人物誤認	Personenverkennung（D），misidentification（E）
人物描画テスト	draw-a-person test（E）
心理教育	psychoeducation（E）
心理緊張	tension psychologique（P. Janet）（F）
心理劇，サイコドラマ	psychodrama（J. L. Moreno）（E）
心理検査	psychological testing（E）
心理自動症	automatisme psychologique（P. Janet）（F）
心理測定	psychometry（E）
心理療法→精神療法	

す

遂行機能	executive function（E）
水頭症*	hydrocephalus（E）
睡眠異常	dyssomnia（E）

睡眠覚醒スケジュール障害	sleep-wake schedule disorder（E）
睡眠過剰	hypersomnia（E）
睡眠驚愕障害	sleep terror disorder（E）
睡眠時随伴症	parasomnia（E）
睡眠（時）てんかん	Schlafepilepsie（D. Janz）（D）
睡眠時無呼吸症候群	sleep apnea syndrome（E）
睡眠時遊行症 ⇒夢遊症	sleepwalking disorder（ICD-10）（E）
睡眠障害	sleep disorder（E）
睡眠潜時反復テスト	multiple sleep latency test（MSLT）（E）
睡眠相後退［遅延］症候群	delayed sleep phase syndrome（E）
睡眠相前進	advanced sleep phase（E）
睡眠導入剤	soporifics（E），Einschlafmittel（D）
睡眠発作	sleep attack（E），Schlafanfall（D）
睡眠麻痺	sleep paralysis（E）
睡眠薬	hypnotics（E）
すくみ足歩行*	frozen gait（E）
スタージ-ウェーバー病*	Sturge-Weber disease（E）
スチューデントアパシー→学生無気力症	
スティグマ，刻印	stigma（E）
捨鉢諧謔，すてばちユーモア	Galgenhumor（D）
ステロイド精神病	steroid psychosis（E）
ストーミー・パーソナリティ	stormy personality（S. Arieti）（E）
ストレス	stress（E）
ストレス因子，ストレッサー	stressor（E）
ストレス脆弱性モデル	vulnerability stress model（E）
スーパーヴィジョン	supervision（E）
スプリッティング	splitting（E）
スペクト→単光子断層撮影	

せ

性格学	characterology（E）
性格神経症	character neurosis（E）
性格変化，人格変化	Charakterveränderung, Persönlichkeitsveränderung（D）
生活指導	guidance of daily activity（E）

生活技能訓練→社会生活技能訓練（法）	
生活史	life history（E）
生活年齢	chronological age（E）
生活の質，クオリティ・オブ・ライフ	quality of life（QOL）（E）
生活保護法	Public Assistance Law（E）
生活療法（小林八郎）	living learning（臺弘）（E）
生活臨床	clinical guidance in way of life（E）
性感帯	erogenous zone（E）
性機能不全（障害）	sexual dysfunction（E）
生気感情	Vitalgefühl（D）
性器期	genital stage（E）
生気抑うつ	vitale Depression（K. Schneider）（D）
生気論	vitalism（E）
性嫌悪障害	sexual aversion disorder（E）
性交疼痛症	dyspareunia（E）
性交疼痛障害	sexual pain disorders（E）
静坐不能，アカシジア	acathisia，akathisia（E）
制止	inhibition（E），Hemmung（D）
正視恐怖→自己視線恐怖	
性嗜好異常→パラフィリア	
静止振戦	resting tremor（E）
正常圧水頭症*	normal pressure hydrocephalus（E）
生殖精神病	Generationspsychose（D）
精神安定薬	tranquilizer（E）
精神医学	psychiatry（E）
精神医学ソーシャルワーカー，精神科ソーシャルワーカー→精神保健福祉士	
精神医学的疫学	psychiatric epidemiology（E）
精神医学的民勢学	psychiatric demography（E）
精神依存	psychic dependence（E）
精神医療審査会	psychiatric review board（E）
精神運動性	Psychomotorik（D）
精神運動（性）興奮	psychomotorishe Erregung（D）
精神運動（性）制止	psychomotorische Hemmung（D）
精神運動発作	psychomotor seizure（E）

精神衛生	mental hygiene（E）
精神我	geistiges Ich（D）
精神科医，精神医学者	psychiatrist（E）
精神解体	désagrégation psychique（F）
精神乖離症（歴史用語）	schizophrenia（E）
精神科看護	psychiatric nursing（E）
精神科救急	emergency psychiatry（E）
精神科クリニック，メンタルクリニック	mental clinic（E）
精神科作業療法	psychiatric occupational therapy（E）
精神（科）病院	mental hospital（E）
精神科病床	psychiatric bed（E）
精神科訪問看護	psychiatric visiting nursing（E）
精神科薬物療法	psychiatric drug therapy（E）
精神科リハビリテーション	psychiatric rehabilitation（E）
精神鑑定	psychiatric evidence，psychiatric testimony（E），psychiatrische Begutachtung，psychiatrisches Gutachten（D），expertise psychiatrique（F）
精神緩慢	bradyphrenia（E）
精神外科	psychosurgery（E）
精神幻覚	hallucination psychique（J. Baillarger）（F）
精神交互作用（森田）	psychic interaction（E）
精神錯乱	confusion mentale（F）
精神作用物質（解説用語）	psychoactive substance（ICD-10）（E）
――依存	substance dependence（DSM-IV）（E）
――関連障害	substance-related disorders（DSM-IV）（E）
――使用障害	substance use disorders（DSM-III）（E）
――中毒	substance intoxication（DSM-IV）（E）
――中毒（性）せん妄	substance intoxication delirium（E）

──誘発（性）障害	substance-induced disorders（DSM-Ⅳ-TR）（E）
──気分障害	substance-induced mood disorder（E）
──睡眠障害	substance-induced sleep disorder（E）
──性機能不全	substance-induced sexual dysfunction（E）
──精神病性障害	substance-induced psychotic disorder（E）
──せん妄	substance-induced delirium（E）
──持続性健忘障害	substance-induced persisting amnestic disorder（E）
──持続性認知［痴呆］症	substance-induced persisting dementia（E）
──不安障害	substance-induced anxiety disorder（E）
──乱用	substance abuse（DSM-Ⅳ）（E）
──離脱	substance withdrawal（DSM-Ⅳ）（E）
──離脱（性）せん妄	substance withdrawal delirium（E）
精神刺激薬	psychostimulant（E）
精神自動症	automatisme mental（G. G. de Clérambault）（F）
精神腫瘍学→サイコオンコロジー	
精神障害	mental disorder（E），Geistesstörung（D），trouble mentale（F）
精神障害者社会適応訓練事業	social adaptation training for the person with mental disorder（E）
精神障害者社会復帰施設	social rehabilitation facility for the person with mental disorder（E）
精神障害者授産施設	sheltered work institution for the person with mental disorder（E）
精神障害者生活訓練施設	facility for training in daily life of the person with mental disorder（E）
精神障害者地域生活援助事業	community life support work for the person with mental disorder（E）

せ

精神障害者地域生活支援センター	community life support center for the person with mental disorder（E）
精神障害者福祉工場	welfare factory for the person with mental disorder（E）
精神障害者福祉ホーム	welfare home for the person with mental disorder（E）
精神障害者保健福祉手帳	certification for health and welfare of the person with mental disorder（E）
精神障害の診断と統計の手引き（アメリカ精神医学会）	Diagnostic and Statistical Manual of Mental Disorders（DSM）（APA）（E）
精神症状評価尺度，病状評価尺度	rating scale for the assesement of psychiatric symptom（E）
精神神経症	psychoneurosis（E）
精神神経免疫	psychoneuroimmunology（E）
精神衰弱	psychasthénie（P. Janet）（F）
精神衰退	mental deterioration（E）
精神性注視麻痺	psychic gaze paralysis（E），Seelenlähmung des Schauens（D）
精神生物学	psychobiology（A. Meyer）（E）
精神生理学	psychophysiology（E）
精神生理性不眠	psychophysiological insomnia（E）
精神測定	psychometry（E）
精神治療学	Seelenheilkunde（D）
精神痛	psychalgia（E）
精神年齢	mental age（MA）（E）
精神薄弱（歴史用語）	mental deficiency，oligophrenia（E），Schwachsinn（D），arriération mentale（F）
精神（発達）遅滞⇒知的障害	mental retardation（E）
軽度精神（発達）遅滞	mild mental retardation（E）
中等度精神（発達）遅滞	moderate mental retardation（E）
重度精神（発達）遅滞	severe mental retardation（E）
最重度精神（発達）遅滞	profound mental retardation（E）
精神反芻→心的反芻	

精神病	psychosis（E）, Psychose（D）, psychose（F）
精神病院法	Mental Hospital Act（E）
精神病後抑うつ	postpsychotic depression（E）
精神病質人格	psychopathische Persönlichkeit（K. Schneider）（D）
精神病者監護法	The Confinement and Protection for Lunatics Act（E）
精神病未治療期間	duration of untreated psychosis（DUP）（E）
精神病理学	psychopathology（E）, Psychopathologie（D）
精神賦活薬	psychic energizer（E）
精神分析	psychoanalysis（E）
精神分裂，精神分裂症（歴史用語）	schizophrenia（E）
精神分裂病（歴史用語）→統合失調症	
精神保健	mental health（E）
精神保健指定医	designated physician of mental health（E）
精神保健センター	mental health center（E）
精神保健福祉士	psychiatric social worker（PSW）（E）
精神保健福祉センター	mental health and welfare center（E）
精神保健福祉法	Mental Health and Welfare Act（E）
精神保健法	Mental Health Law（E）
精神発作	psychic seizure（W. G. Lennox）, psychical seizure（W. Penfield）（E）
精神免疫学	psychoimmunology（E）
精神盲	Seelenblindheit（D）
精神薬理学	psychopharmacology（E）
精神力動	psychodynamics（E）
精神療法，心理療法	psychotherapy（E）
精神聾	Seelentaubheit（D）
精神論者	Psychiker（D）
正染性白質ジストロフィー*	orthochromatic leukodystrophy（E）
性的虐待	sexual abuse（E）

性的興奮の障害	sexual arousal disorder（E）
性的サディズム	sexual sadism（E）
性的神経衰弱	sexual neurasthenia（E）
性的早熟	prematura sexualis, pubertas praecox（L）
性的反応不全	failure of genital response（E）
性的不能症, インポテンツ	impotence（E）
性的マゾヒズム	sexual masochism（E）
性的欲求低下障害	hypoactive sexual desire disorder（E）
静的了解	statisches Verstehen（D）
性転換症	transsexualism（E）
性（別）同一性	gender identity（E）
性同一性障害	gender identity disorder（E）
性倒錯	sexual perversion（E）
青年期	adolescence（E）
成年後見	adult guardianship（E）
成年後見制度	adult guardian system（E）
青年（期）精神医学	adolescent psychiatry（E）
制縛神経症	anancastic neurosis（E）
制縛（性）パーソナリティ［人格］障害 ⇒強迫性パーソナリティ［人格］障害	anancastic personality disorder（E）
性不感症	sexual frigidity（E）
生物学的精神医学	biological psychiatry（E）
性欲過剰, 性欲亢進	hypersexuality（E）
性欲減退	hyposexuality（E）
世界精神医学会	World Psychiatric Association（WPA）（E）
世界没落体験	Weltuntergangserlebnis（D）
脊髄癆進行麻痺	taboparesis, taboparalysis（E）, Taboparalyse（D）
責任能力	criminal responsibility（E）, Schuldfähigkeit（D）
責任無能力	lack of criminal responsibility（E）, Schuldunfähigkeit（D）
赤面恐怖	ereuthophobia, erythrophobia（E）

セクシュアル・ハラスメント	sexual harassment（E）
石灰沈着を伴うびまん性神経原線維変化症	diffuse neurofibrillary tangles with calcification（DNTC）（E）
窃視（症）	voyeurism（E），Schaulust（D）
接枝統合失調症	Propfschizophrenie（D），graft schizophrenia（E）
接枝破瓜病	Propfhebephrenie（D）
接触	contact（E）
摂食障害	eating disorder（E）
絶体臥褥期（森田療法）	absolute bedrest（Morita therapy）（E）
窃盗恐怖	cleptophobia（E）
説得療法	persuasion therapy（E）
説明と承諾**（解説用語）→インフォームド・コンセント	
説明妄想（解説用語）	Erklärungswahn（C. Wernicke）（D），explanatory delusion（E）
セネストパチー→体感症	
セルフヘルプグループ→自助グループ	
セロトニン・ドパミン遮断薬	serotonin-dopamine inhibitor（E）
セロトニン・ノルアドレナリン再取り込み阻害薬	serotonin-noradrenaline reuptake inhibitor（SNRI）（E）
前意識の	preconscious（E）
線維束攣縮*	fasciculation（E）
線維攣縮*	fibrillation（E）
遷延（性）うつ病	prolonged depression（E）
閃輝暗点	scintillating scotoma（E）
前駆期統合失調症	prodromal schizophrenia（E）
前駆状態	prodromal state（E）
前屈小発作	Propulsiv-Petit mal（D. Janz）（D）
全健忘	total amnesia（E）
前向健忘	anterograde amnesia（E）
全国精神障害者家族会連合会（全家連）	National Federation of Families with Mentaly Ill in Japan（E）

全国精神保健福祉会連合会	National Federation of Mental Health and Welfare Party in Japan："Minna Net"（E）
潜在期，潜伏期	latency period（E），Latenzperiode（D）
潜在記憶⇒顕在記憶	cryptomnesia（E），cryptomnesie（T. Flournoy）（F）
潜在統合失調症	latent schizophrenia（E）
潜在統合失調症様反応	latent schizophreniform reaction（E）
せんさく癖	Grübelsucht（D）
全失語	global aphasia, total aphasia（E）
洗浄強迫	washing compulsion（E），Waschenzwang（D）
線条体黒質変性症*	striatonigral degeneration（SND）（E）
全生活史健忘	amnesia of personal history（E），allgemeine Amnesie（D）
前性器期	pregenital stage（E）
前精神病期	prepsychotic stage（E）
戦争神経症	Kriegsneurose（D）
全体感情妄想	holothymer Wahn（D）
全体障害	Ganzheitsstörung（D）
全体論	holism（E）
選択緘黙症，選択無言症	elective mutism, selective mutism（E），mutisme electif（F），elektiver Mutismus（M. Tramer）（D）
選択健忘	selective amnesia（E），amnésie élective（F）
選択的セロトニン再取り込み阻害薬	selective serotonin reuptake inhibitor（SSRI）（E）
選択的不注意	selective inattention（H. S. Sullivan）（E）
先端恐怖	aichmophobia（E）
前兆，アウラ	aura（E）
前頭側頭型認知［痴呆］症	frontotemporal dementia（FTD）（E）
前頭側頭葉変性症	frontotemporal lobar degeneration（FTLD）（E）

前頭葉機能低下	hypofrontality（E）
前頭葉症候群	frontal lobe syndrome（E）, Stirnhirnsyndrom（D）
前頭葉ロボトミー	frontal lobotomy（W. Freeman & J. W. Watts）（E）
洗脳	brain wash（E）
全能感	feeling of omnipotence（E）, Allmachtsgefühl（D）
全般けいれん発作	generalized convulsive seizure（E）
全般性不安障害	generalized anxiety disorder（E）
全般てんかん	generalized epilepsy（E）
潜伏統合失調症	latent schizophrenia（E）
前部前頭葉白質切截術	prefrontal leucotomy（E. Moniz）（E）
せん妄	delirium（E）

そ

素因	predisposition（E）
躁うつ病	manic-depressive psychosis（E）, manisch-depressive Irresein（D）, psychose maniaco-dépressive（F）
挿間性もうろう状態	episodischer Dämmerzustand（D）
想起→再生	
早期精神病	early psychosis（E）
早期幼児自閉症⇒自閉症	early infantile autism（L. Kanner）（E）
双極Ⅰ型障害	bipolar I disorder（DSM-Ⅳ-TR）（E）
双極Ⅱ型障害	bipolar II disorder（DSM-Ⅳ-TR）（E）
双極うつ病	bipolar depression（E）
双極感情障害	bipolar affective disorder（E）
双極（性）障害	bipolar disorder（DSM-Ⅳ-TR）（E）
造語（症）→言語新作	
総合病院精神医学	general hospital psychiatry（E）
蒼古的	archaic（E）
操作（的）診断（学）	operation diagnosis（E）
早産児	preterm infant（E）
層次神経症	Schichtneurose（J. H. Schultz）（D）

巣症状	focal symptom（E），Herdsymptom（D）
層診断	Schichtdiagnose（D）
双生児研究	twin study（E）
想像界	l'imaginaire（J. Lacan）（F）
創造の病	maladie créatrice（H. F. Ellenberger）（F）
早朝覚醒	early morning awakening（E）
躁的防衛	manic defense（E）
躁転	manic switch（E）
早発痴呆（歴史用語）（解説用語）	dementia praecox（E. Kraepelin）（L）
躁病	mania（E），Manie（D），manie（F）
躁病エピソード	manic episode（DSM-IV-TR）（E）
相貌学	Physiognomik（D）
相貌失認	prosopagnosia（E）
層理論	Schichtentheorie（D），stratification theory（E）
早漏	premature ejaculation（E）
挿話，エピソード	episode（E）
疎遠，疎隔	Entfremdung（D）
疎隔感	Entfremdungsgefühl（D）
即時記憶	immediate memory（E）
測定障害*	dysmetria（E）
側頭葉てんかん	temporal lobe epilepsy（E）
続発てんかん	secondary epilepsy（E）
素行および情動の混在性障害	mixed disorder of conduct and emotion（ICD-10）（E）
素行障害（解説用語）	conduct disorder（DSM-III）（E）
措置入院	involuntary hospitalization ordered by prefectural governor（E）
疎通性	accessibility（E），Zugänglichkeit（D）
ソンディテスト	Szondi test（E）

た

体因性	somatogenic（E）
大うつ病	major depression（DSM-III）（E）

大うつ病性障害	major depressive disorder（DSM-IV）（E）
体液（病理）説	humoral pathology（E），Humoralpathologie（D）
怠学	school truancy（E）
体感	cénesthésie（F）
体感異常型統合失調症	coenästhetische Schizophrenie（G. Huber）（D）
体感症，セネストパチー	cénestopathie（F），cenesthopathy（E）
体系妄想，系統妄想	systematischer Wahn（D），systematized delusion（E）
体験加工	Erlebnisverarbeitung（D）
体験反応	Erlebnisreaktion（D）
退行	regression（E）
退行期うつ病，退行期メランコリー（解説用語）	involutional melancholia（E），Involutionsmelancholie（D）
退行期精神病	involutional psychosis（E）
対抗強迫	Gegenzwang（D）
対抗転移→逆転移	
対光反射*	light reflex（E）
太古思想	archaisches Denken（D）
胎児（性）アルコール症候群	fetal alcohol syndrome（E）
胎児姿勢	Embryonalstellung（D）
大視症	macropsia（E）
大字症	macrographia（E）
体臭恐怖→自己臭恐怖	
対処（行動）→コーピング	
対象意識	Gegenstandsbewußtsein（D）
帯状回発作	cingulate seizure（E）
対象関係論	object relations theory（E）
対象喪失	object loss（E）
対象リビド	object libido（E）
大食（症），過食（症）	bulimia（E）
対人恐怖（症）⇒交際恐怖	anthropophobia（E）
耐性	tolerance（E）

胎生期	fetal period（E）
滞続談話，滞続言語	stehende Redensart（D）
大頭症*	macrocephaly，megacephaly（E）
第二世代抗精神病薬	second generation antipsychotics（SGA）（E）
大脳局在論	theory of cerebral localization（E），Lokalisationslehre（D）
大脳側性化	cerebral lateralization（E）
大脳半球優位	cerebral dominance（E）
大脳半球離断症候群	cerebral hemisphere disconnection［disconnexion］syndrome（E）
大脳皮質基底核変性症*	corticobasal degeneration（CBD）（E）
大脳辺縁系	limbic system（E）
大ヒステリー	grand hystérie（J. M. Charcot）（F）
大発作	generalized convalsion（E），grand mal（F）
大麻	cannabis（E）
——依存	cannabis dependence（E）
——関連障害	cannabis-related disorders（E）
——中毒	cannabis intoxication（E）
——中毒せん妄	cannabis intoxication delirium（E）
——誘発性障害	cannabis-induced disorders（E）
——乱用	cannabis abuse（E）
怠薬⇒ノンコンプライアンス	
退薬→離脱	
代理形成	substitution，substitutive formation（E），Ersatzbildung（D）
代理ミュンヒハウゼン症候群	Munchausen syndrome by proxy（E）
多因子遺伝，ポリジーン遺伝	polygene inheritance（E）
タウ蛋白*	tau protein（E）
タウオパチー*，タウ異常症*	tauopathy（E）
ダウン症候群	Down syndrome（E）
ダウンレギュレーション，下向調節	down regulation（E）
妥協形成	compromise formation（E）
多棘複合	multiple spike complex（E）

多系統萎縮症*	multiple system atrophy（MSA）（E）
多元診断	mehrdimensionale Diagnostik（E. Kretschmer）（D）, multidimensional diagnosis（E）
多幸症，上機嫌症	euphoria（E）
多軸評価	multiaxial evaluation（E）
多重人格	multiple personality（E）
多重人格障害	multiple personality disorder（ICD-10, DSM-III-R）（E）
多食（症）	polyphagia（E）
多精神作用物質依存	polysubstance dependence（DSM-III-R）（E）
多精神作用物質関連障害	polysubstance-related disorder（DSM-IV）（E）
立ちなおり反射*	righting reflex（E）
脱感作療法	desensitization therapy（E）
脱施設化	deinstitutionalization（E）
脱神経*	denervation（E）
脱髄疾患*	demyelinating disease（E）
脱抑制→抑制消失	
脱抑制性愛着障害	disinhibited attachment disorder（E）
脱力発作，カタプレキシー	cataplexy（E）
多動（症）	hyperkinesis（E）
多動（性）障害	hyperkinetic disorder（ICD-10）（E）
田中-ビネ式知能検査，田中-ビネ法	Tanaka-Binet test（E）
ターナー症候群	Turner syndrome（E）
煙草依存⇒ニコチン依存	tobacco dependance（DSM-III）（E）
多発棘波	polyspikes（E）
多発（性）硬化症*	multiple sclerosis（MS）（E）
多発梗塞（性）認知［痴呆］症	multi-infarct dementia（E）
多発神経炎精神病→コルサコフ精神病	psychose polynervritique（F）
ダブルバインド説，二重拘束説	double bind theory（G. Bateson）（E）
多文化間精神医学	transcultural psychiatry（E）
ターミナルケア，終末医療	terminal care（E）

単一精神病	Einheitspsychose（W. Griesinger, H. W. Neuman）（D）
短期記憶	short term memory（E）
短期精神病性障害	brief psychotic disorder（DSM-IV）（E）
短期精神療法	short-term psychotherapy（E）
短期反応（性）精神病	brief reactive psychosis（DSM-III）（E）
単極（性）うつ病	unipolar depression（E），monopolare Depression（D）
単光子断層撮影，スペクト	single photon emission computed tomography（SPECT）（E）
男根期	phallic stage（E）
短時間睡眠者	short sleeper（E）
断酒会	temperance society（E）
単純型統合失調症	simple schizophrenia, schizophrenia, simple type（E）
単純（型）荒廃性障害	simple deteriorative disorder（E）
単純痴呆（歴史用語）	dementia simplex（L）
単純ヘルペス脳炎＊	herpes simplex encephalitis（E）
単純酩酊	simple drunkenness（E）
男性化	masculinization（E）
男性色情症	satyriasis（E）
断綴言語，断綴性発語＊	scanning speech（E）
断眠	sleep deprivation（E）
短絡反応	Kurzschlußreaktion（D），short circuit reaction（E）
談話心迫	Rededrang（D）

ち

地域精神医学	community psychiatry（E）
地域組織化	community organization（E）
地域福祉権利擁護事業	advocacy for community welfare（E）
遅延反響言語	delayed echolalia（E）
知覚抗争（井村恒郎）	perceptual rivalry（E）
知覚消去＊→感覚消去	

知覚変容	sensory distortion, perceptual alteration（E）
致死（性）緊張病	tödliche Katatonie（K. H. Stauder）（D）, lethal catatonia（E）
地誌的記憶障害	topographical dysmnesia（E）
知性化	intellectualization（E）
知性精神	Noopsyche（E. Stransky）（D）
チック	tic（E）
チック障害	tic disorder（ICD-10, DSM-III）（E）
膣けいれん	vaginismus（E）
知的障害（解説用語）	mental retardation（E）
知的障害援護施設（解説用語）	support institusion for intellectually disorder（E）
知能	intelligence（E）, Intelligenz（D）
知能検査	intelligence test（E）, Intelligenzprüfung（D）
知能指数	intelligence quotient（IQ）（E）
知能年齢	Intelligenzalter（D）
遅発（性）うつ病	late depression（E）, Spätdepression（D）
遅発（性）緊張病	Spätkatatonie（M. Sommer）（D）, late catatonia（E）
遅発（性）ジスキネジー［ジスキネジア］	tardive dyskinesia（E）
遅発（性）てんかん	Spätepilepsie（D）
遅発（性）統合失調症	late schizophrenia（E）, Spätschizophrenie（D）
遅発（性）パラフレニー［パラフレニア］	late paraphrenia（M. Roth）（E）
痴呆（症）→認知症	
地方精神保健福祉審議会	local council on mental health and welfare（E）
着衣失行	apraxia for dressing, dressing apraxia（E）, Kleidungsapraxie, Bekleidungsapraxie（D）
注意欠如障害	attention deficit disorder（ADD）（DSM-III）（E）

注意欠如・多動（性）障害	attention-deficit/hyperactivity disorder (ADHD)（DSM-IV）（E）
――混合型	combined type（E）
――多動性-衝動性優勢型	predominantly hyperactive-impulsive type（E）
――不注意優勢型	predominantly inattentive type（E）
注意減弱，注意減退	hypoprosexia（E）
中核神経症	Kernneurose（J. H. Schultz）（D）
昼間遺尿（症）	enuresis diurnal（L），diurnal enuresis（E）
中間施設	transitional facility（E）
昼間病院⇒デイホスピタル	
注察妄想	delusion of observation（E），Beachtungswahn，Beobachtungswahn（D）
中軸症状	axial symptom（E），Achsensymptom（D）
注視けいれん	Blickkrampf（D）
注視発作⇒眼球回転発作	oculogyric crisis（E），Blickanfall，Schauanfall（D）
抽象的態度	abstraktes Verhalten（K. Goldstein）（D），abstract attitude（E）
中心側頭部脳波焦点良性小児てんかん	benign epilepsy of children with centro-temporal EEG foci（BECCT）（E）
中心脳発作	centrencephalic seizure（E）
中枢刺激薬	psychostimulant（E）
中枢神経梅毒*	neurosyphilis（E）
中等度精神（発達）遅滞	moderate mental retardation（E）
中途覚醒	intermittent awakening（E）
中毒（性）精神病	intoxication psychosis（E），Intoxikationspsychose（D）
中脳幻覚症	hallucinose pédonculaire（J. Lhermitte）（F）
聴唖	Hörstummheit（D）

超越論的現象学	transzendentale Phänomenologie (E. Husserl)（D）
聴覚失認	auditory agnosia（E）
聴覚発作	auditory seizure（E）
長期記憶	long term memory（E）
聴原発作	auditogenic seizure（E）
（超）高齢化社会	aged society（E）
超自我	super-ego（E），Über-Ich（D）
調節反射*	accommodation reflex（E）
腸内寄生虫妄想	Enterozoenwahn（D）
超皮質（性）失語（症）	transcortical aphasia（E），transkortikale Aphasie（D）
──運動失語（症）	transcortical motor aphasia（E）
──感覚失語（症）	transcortical sensory aphasia（E）
重複記憶錯誤	reduplicating paramnesia（E）
直観像素質	eidetische Anlage（E. R. Jaensch）（D）
直観像素質者	Eidetiker（E. R. Jaensch）（D）
治療を受ける権利	right of treatment（E）
治療を拒否する権利	right to refuse treatment（E）
治療可能な認知［痴呆］症	treatable dementia（E）
治療教育	educational treatment, remedial education（E），Heilpädagogik（D）
治療共同体，治療共同社会	therapeutic community（E）
治療契約	therapeutic contract（E）
治療構造	structure of psychotherapy（E）
治療・服薬遵守不良→ノンコンプライアンス	
治療的退行	therapeutic regression（E）
治療同盟	therapeutic alliance（E）
陳述記憶，宣言記憶	declarative memory（E）

つ

追想幻覚	Erinnerungshalluzination（D）
追想錯覚	Erinnerungsillusion（D）

つ〜て

追想錯誤	Erinnerungsfälschung（D）, Erinnerungstäuschung（D）
痛覚失象徴	Schmerzasymbolie（D）, asymbolia for pain（E）
通過儀礼	initiation ceremony（E）
通過症候群	Durchgangssyndrom（H. H. Wieck）（D）, transit syndrome（E）
つぎ足歩行*	tandem gait（E）
つきもの妄想→憑依妄想	
償い，修復作用	reparation（M. Klein）（E）, Wiedergutmachung（D）
つまずき言葉*	Silbenstolpern（D）
爪かみ	nail biting, onchophagia（E）

て

ディアシージス	Diaschisis（C. v. Monakow）（D）
デイケア	day care（E）
抵抗症*	Gegenhalten（D）, paratonic rigidity（E）
抵抗分析	Widerstandanalyse（S. Freud）（D）, resistance analysis（E）
停止型進行麻痺	stationary paresis, arrested paresis（E）, stationäre Paralyse（D）
停止発作	arrest seizure（E）
デイホスピタル	day hospital（E）
適応障害	adjustment disorder（ICD-10, DSM-III）（E）
出来事的記憶→エピソード記憶	
テクノストレス	technostress（E）
手首自傷→リストカット	
手続き記憶	procedural memory（E）
徹底操作	Durcharbeitung（S. Freud）（D）, working throuth（E）
鉄道脊椎症*	railway spine（E）
でまかせ応答→的はずし応答	

テレパシー	telepathy（E）
転移	Übertragung（D），transference（E），transfert（F）
転換	conversion（E）
てんかん	epilepsy（E），Epilepsie（D），épilepsie（F）
てんかん学	epileptology（E）
てんかん重積状態，てんかん発作重積	status epilepticus（L）
転換性障害	conversion disorder（ICD-10，DSM-III）（E）
てんかん（性）精神病	epileptic psychosis（E）
転換ヒステリー	conversion hysteria（E）
てんかん病質（歴史用語）	epileptoid（E），Epileptoid（D）
てんかん発作（性）昏迷	ictal stupor（E）
てんかん（性）もうろう状態	epileptic twilight state（E），epileptischer Dämmerzustand（D）
電気けいれん療法，通電療法	electroconvulsive treatment, electroconvulsive therapy（ECT）（E）
電気ショック療法	Elektroschocktherapie（ES）（D）
電撃・点頭・礼拝けいれん	Blitz-Nick-Salaam Krampf（B-N-S Krampf）（D）
伝達可能な認知［痴呆］症	transmissible dementia（E）
伝導失語（症）	conduction aphasia（E）
転導性	distractibility（E），Ablenkbarkeit（D）
点頭てんかん	infantile spasms（F. A. &E. L. Gibbs）（E）

と

当意即答→的はずし応答	
同一化，同一視	identification（E）
同一性拡散症候群	identity diffusion syndrome（E. H. Erikson）（E）
同一性危機	identity crisis（E. H. Erikson）（E）
頭位めまい*	positional vertigo（E）

動因喪失症候群	amotivational syndrome（E）
投影，投射	projection（E），Projektion（D）
投影による同一視	projective identification（M. Klein）（E）
投影［映］法，	projective method（E）
盗害妄想，もの盗られ妄想	delusion of robbery（E），Bestehlungswahn（D）
統覚	apperception（E）
等価症	equivalent（E）
同期（性）	synchrony, synchronous（E）
冬季うつ病	winter depression（E）
動機づけ	motivation（E）
道具障害	Werkzeugstörung（D）
道具の強迫的使用現象	compulsive manipulation of tools（E）
道化症候群	buffoonery syndrome（E），Faxensyndrom（D）
統合教育	integrated education（E）
登校拒否	school refusal（E）
頭後屈反射*	head retraction reflex（E）
統合失調型障害	schizotypal disorder（ICD-10）（E）
統合失調型パーソナリティ［人格］障害	schizotypal personality disorder（DSM-III）（E）
統合失調感情障害	schizo-affective disorder（ICD-10, DSM-III）（E）
統合失調感情精神病	schizo-affective psychosis（J. Kassanin）（E）
統合失調気質，スキゾサイミア	schizothymia（E）
統合失調言語（症）	schizophasia（E）
統合失調質，スキゾイド	schizoid（E）
統合失調質パーソナリティ［人格］障害	schizoid personality disorder（ICD-10, DSM-III）（E）
統合失調症	schizophrenia（E），Schizophrenie（D）
統合失調症後抑うつ	postschizophrenic depression（E）
統合失調症性認知［痴呆］症	schizophrenic dementia（E）
統合失調症性反応	schizophrenic reaction（E）

統合失調症様障害	schizophreniform disorder（DSM-Ⅲ）（E）
統合失調症様精神病	schizophreniform psychosis（G. Langfeldt）（E）
統合失調症をつくる母	schizophrenogenic mother（F. Fromm=Reichmann）（E）
瞳孔不同*	anisocoria（E）
同語反復	palilalia（E）
動作振戦*	action tremor（E）
動作性知能指数	performance intelligence quotient（PIQ）（E）
洞察	insight（E），Einsicht（D）
洞察療法	insight therapy（E）
闘士型	athletic（E）
同時失認	simultanagnosia（E），Simultanagnosie（D）
島失語	island aphasia（E），Inselaphasie（D）
同性愛	homosexuality（E）
同席精神療法	conjoint psychotherapy（E）
同席面接	joint interview（E）
闘争パラノイア，闘争妄想（症）	Kampfparanoia（D）
同調性	syntone（E），Synton（D）
疼痛恐怖（症）	algophobia（E）
疼痛（性）障害	pain disorder（DSM-Ⅳ）（E）
疼痛性愛	algomania, algolagnia（E）
動的家族描画法	kinetic family drawing（KFD）（E）
道徳療法→モラル療法	
逃避	escape（E），Flucht（D）
動物恐怖（症）	zoophobia（E）
動物幻視	zoopsia（E）
動物磁気，生動磁気（歴史用語）	magnétisme animal（F），animal magnetism（E）
動物性愛	zoophilia（E）
盗癖	cleptomania（E），Stehltrieb（D）
同胞葛藤，同胞抗争	sibling rivalry（E）

同胞葛藤（性）障害，同胞抗争（性）障害	sibling rivalry disorder（ICD-10）（E）
同名半盲*	homonymous hemianopsia（E）
トゥレット症候群，ジル・ドゥ・ラ・トゥレット症候群	Tourette syndrome, Gilles de la Tourette Syndrome（E）
当惑作話	Verlegenheitskonfabulation（D）
とがり口	Schnauzkrampf（D）
トキソプラスマ症*	toxoplasmosis（E）
特異的会話構音障害	specific speech articulation disorder（ICD-10）（E）
特異的算数能力障害	specific disorder of arithmetical skills（ICD-10）（E）
特異的綴字障害	specific spelling disorder（ICD-10）（E）
特異的読字障害	specific reading disorder（ICD-10）（E）
特異的発達障害	specific developmental disorder（ICD-10, DSM-III）（E）
独語	monolog(ue)（E）, Selbstgespräch（D）
読字障害	dyslexia（E）
特殊教育	special education（E）
読書障害，読字障害	reading disorder（ICD-10, DSM-III）（E）
読書遅滞	reading retardation（ICD-9）（E）
読書てんかん	reading epilepsy（E）
読書反響	écho de la lecture（F）
特別養護老人ホーム	nursing home for the aged under poor conditions（E）
匿名断酒会→アルコール患者匿名会	
閉じこめ症候群*	locked-in syndrome（E）
途絶	blocking（E）, Sperrung（D）
突発性律動異常波	paroxysmal dysrhythmia（E）
塗糞	Kotschmieren（D）
トラウマ→心的外傷	

とらわれ（森田療法）	mental preoccupation（Morita therapy）（E）
トランス	trance（E）
取り入れ	introjection（E），Introjektion（D）
取り消し，打ち消し	undoing（E），Ungeschehenmachen（S. Freud）（D）
遁走，フーグ	fugue（E，F）

な

内因（性）	endogenous（E）
――うつ病	endogenous depression（E）
――精神病	endogenous psychosis（E）
内因反応性気分変調（症）	endoreaktive Dysthymie（H. J. Weitbrecht）（D）
内界意識	Autopsyche（C. Wernicke）（D）
内観療法	Naikan therapy（E）
内言語	inner speech（E）
内向	introversion（E）
内示記憶	implicit memory（E）
内省	introspection（E），Selbstreflexion（D）
ナイトホスピタル	night hospital（E）
内分泌精神医学	endocrinological psychiatry（E）
内分泌精神症候群	endokrines Psychosyndrom（M. Bleuler）（D）
ナラティブ医学	narrative based medicine（E）
ナルシ（シ）スム→自己愛	
ナルコレプシー	narcolepsy（E）
喃語	babbling（E）
難治（性）うつ病	intractable depression（E）

に

荷おろしうつ病	Entlastungsdepression（W. Schulte）（D）
肉体的虐待→身体的虐待	

ニコチン依存	nicotine dependence（DSM-III-R）（E）
ニコチン関連障害	nicotine-related disorder（DSM-IV）（E）
二語文	two-word sentence（E）
二次妄想	secondary delusion（E），sekundärer Wahn（D）
二次利得	secondary gain（E）
二重化体験	Verdoppelungserlebnis（D）
二重見当識，二重定位	double orientation（E），doppelte Orientierung（D）
二重拘束，ダブルバインド	double bind（G. Bateson）（E）
二重思考	Doppeldenken（D）
二重身，ドッペルゲンガー	Doppelgänger（D）
二重人格	double personality（E），doppelte Persönlichkeit（D）
日内変動	daily fluctuation，diurnal fluctuation（E），Tagesschwankung（D）
日本精神科病院協会	Japanese Association of Psychiatric Hospitals（E）
日本精神神経科診療所協会	Japanese Association of Neuro-Psychiatric Clinics（E）
日本精神神経学会	Japanese Society of Psychiatry and Neurology（JSPN）（E）
日本精神保健福祉連盟	Japan Federation for Mental Health and Welfare（E）
日本脳炎	japanese encephalitis（E），encephalitis japonica（L）
ニーマン-ピック病*	Niemann-Pick disease（E）
入院患者	inpatient（E）
乳児院	infant home（E）
乳頭浮腫*→うっ血乳頭*	
入眠幻覚	hypnagogic hallucination（E）
入眠困難，就眠困難	difficulty of falling asleep（E）
入眠潜時反復テスト	multiple sleep latency test（MSLT）（E）

入眠体験	Einschlaferlebnis（D）
乳幼児けいれん	infantile convulsion（E）
乳幼児精神医学	infantile psychiatry（E）
任意後見制度	voluntary guardianship system（E）
任意症状	facultive symptom（E）
任意入院	voluntary hospitalization（E）
人形の目現象（反射，試験，徴候）＊	doll's eye phenomenon（reflex, test, sign）（E）
妊娠精神病	Schwangerschaftspsychose（D）
認知症，痴呆（症）	dementia（E），Demenz（D），démence（F）
認知障害	cognitive deficit（E）
認知心理学	cognitive psychology（E）
認知療法	cognitive therapy（E）
ニンフォマニア	nymphomania（E）

ぬ

ヌミノーゼ	Numinose（R. Otto）（D）

ね

根こ（そ）ぎうつ病	Entwurzelungsdepression（H. Bürger-Prinz）（D）
熱（性）けいれん	febrile convulsion（E）
熱情精神病	psychose passionnelle（G. G. de Clérambault）（F）
熱（性）せん妄	Fieberdelirium（D）
寝ぼけ	excessive sleepness（E），Schlaftrunkenheit（D）
年金神経症	Pensionsneurose（D）
粘着（性）気質	visköses Temperament（E. Kretschmer），Kollathymie（W. Enke）（D）
粘着性	viscosity（E）

の

脳炎	encephalitis（E）
脳器質精神症候群	organisches Psychosyndrom（M. Bleuler）（D）
脳局所精神症候群	hirnlokales Psychosyndrom（M. Bleuler）（D）
脳空洞症→孔脳症*	
脳血管性うつ病→血管性うつ病	
脳血管性頭痛→血管性頭痛	
脳血管性認知［痴呆］症→血管性認知［痴呆］症	
脳挫傷	brain contusion（E）
脳死	brain death（E）
脳磁図	magnetoencephalography（MEG）（E）
脳写	encephalography（E）
脳震盪	brain concussion（E）
脳震盪後症候群	postconcussion syndrome（ICD-10）（E）
脳震盪精神病	Kommotionspsychose（D）
脳性麻痺	cerebral palsy（E），zerebrale Kinderlähmung（D）
脳卒中後うつ病	poststroke depression（E）
脳地図	map of cerebral cortex（E），Gehirnkarte（D）
能動（性）意識	Aktivitätsbewußtsein（D）
能動性欠乏	Aktivitätsmangel（D）
脳動脈硬化（症）	cerebral arteriosclerosis（E），Hirnarteriosklerose（D）
脳波	electroencephalogram, electroencephalography（EEG）（E）
脳梅毒	cerebral syphilis（E），Hirnlues（D）
脳波トポグラフィー	EEG topography（E）
脳病理学	brain pathology（E），Gehirnpathologie（D）
脳浮腫*	cerebral edema（E）

脳梁欠損*	agenesis of corpus callosum, callosal agenesis（E）, Balkenmangel（D）
脳梁失行	Balkenapraxie（D）
脳梁症候群	corpus callosum syndrome（E）
ノーマライゼーション	normalization（E）
乗物恐怖（症）	amaxophobia（E）
ノンコンプライアンス，治療・服薬遵守不良，怠薬	non-compliance（E）
ノンレム睡眠	non-REM sleep（E）

は

把握反射*	grasp reflex（E）, Greifreflex（D）
バイオフィードバック療法	bio-feedback therapy（E）
徘徊自動症，歩行（性）自動症	automatisme ambulatoire（F）, ambulatory automatism（E）
徘徊癖	pariomania, dromomania（E）, Wandersucht（D）
配偶者間暴力	violence by partner（E）
背景反応	Hintergrundreaktion（D）
賠償神経症	compensation neurosis（E）, Rentenneurose（D）
排泄訓練，トイレットトレーニング	toilet training（E）
梅毒恐怖（症）	syphilophobia（E）
バウムテスト，樹木画テスト	tree test（E）, Baumtest（D）
破壊的行動障害	distructive behavier disorder（E）
破瓜型統合失調症	hebephrenic schizophrenia, schizophrenia hebephrenic type（E）
破瓜病	Hebephrenie（E. Hecker）（D）, hebephrenia（E）
歯ぎしり	gnash（E）, Zahnknirschen（G）
破局反応	Katastrophenreaktion（K. Goldstein）（D）
パーキンソン症候群	Parkinsonian syndrome, Parkinsonism（E）

パーキンソン認知［痴呆］症複合	Parkinson-dementia complex, Parkinsonism-dementia complex（E）
パーキンソン病*	Parkinson disease（E）
迫害妄想→被害妄想	
白日夢	day dream（E），Tagtraum（D）
爆発型（精神病質者）	Explosible（Psychopathen）（K. Schneider）（D）
歯車固縮*	cogwheel rigidity（E）
箱庭療法	sand play（E），Sandspiel（D）
はさみ（脚）歩行*	scissors gait（E）
パーシャルアゴニスト，部分作動物質［薬］	partial agonist（E）
場所失見当（識）	spatial disorientation（E），örtliche Desorientiertheit（D）
長谷川式簡易知能評価スケール	Hasegawa Dementia Scale（HDS，改訂版 HDS-R）（E）
パーソナリティ，人格	personality（E）
パターナリズム	paternalism（E）
発語緩慢*	bradylalia（E）
発生的了解	genetisches Verstehen（D）
発生率	incidence（E）
発達課題	developmental task（E）
発達（性）協調運動障害	developmental coordination disorder（DSM-III-R）（E）
発達検査	developmental test（E）
発達（性）構音障害	developmental ariculation disorder（DSM-III）（E）
発達指数	developmental quotient（DQ）（E）
発達（性）失語（症）	developmental aphasia（E）
発達（性）失読失書	developmental alexia and agraphia（E）
発達（性）障害	developmental disorder（E）
発達障害［発達能力低下］支援法	Law for Supporting Persons with Developmental Disabilities（E）
発達診断	developmental diagnosis（E）
発達年齢	developmental age（E）

発動（性）失行（症）	Antriebsapraxie（D）
発動性	impulse（E），Antrieb（D）
発動性欠乏	Antriebsmangel（D）
（発）熱療法	fever therapy（E），Fiebertherapie（D）
発明妄想	delusion of invention（E），Erfindungswahn（D）
抜毛癖	trichotillomania（E）
発揚型（精神病質者）	Hyperthymische（Psychopathen）（K. Schneider）（D）
パニック障害	panic disorder（ICD-10，DSM-III-R）（E）
パニック発作	panic attack（DSM-III）（E）
羽ばたき振戦*	flapping tremor（E）
ハビリテーション	habilitation（E）
ハーフウェイハウス，中間施設	halfway house（E）
ハミルトンうつ病評価尺度	Hamilton Rating Scale for Depression（E）
場面無言（症），場面緘黙（症）	situational mutism（E）
早口言語症，乱雑言語症	cluttering（E）
パラソムニア	parasomnia（E）
パラタクシックな歪み	parataxic distortion（H. S. Sullivan）（E）
パラトニー*	paratonia，paratony（E），Gegenhalten（D）
パラノイア，妄想症	paranoia（E）
パラノイド・スキゾイド態勢	paranoid-schizoid position（E）
パラフィリア	paraphilia（E）
パラフレニー	paraphrenia（E）
バリズム*	ballism（E）
バーリント症候群	Bálint syndrome（E）
パレイドリア，変像（症）	pareidoria（E）
反響言語	echolalia（E）
反響症状	echo symptom（E）
反響動作	echopraxia（E）
反響表情	echomimia（E）
反抗期	period of opposition（E）

反抗挑戦性障害	oppositional defiant disorder（DSM-IV）（E）
犯罪精神医学	criminal psychiatry（E）
反社会(性)パーソナリティ[人格]障害	antisocial personality disorder（DSM-III）（E）
反射幻覚	reflex hallucination（E）
反射てんかん	reflex epilepsy（E）
反芻(性)障害	rumination disorder（DSM-III）（E）
反精神医学	antipsychiatry（E）
半側空間失認	unilateral spatial agnosia（E）
半側空間無視	unilateral spatial neglect（E）
半側身体失認	hemiasomatognosia（E）
範疇的態度	kategoriales Verhalten（K. Goldstein）（D），categorical attitude（E）
反跳性不眠	rebound insomnia（E）
ハンチントン病*	Huntington disease（E）
ハンディキャップ→社会的不利	
汎適応症候群	general adaptation syndrome（H. Selye）（E）
反動形成	reaction formation（E），Reaktionsbildung（D）
反応(性)うつ病，反応(性)抑うつ	reactive depression（E）
反応(性)健忘	reactive amnesia（E）
反応(性)興奮	reactive excitement（E）
反応性愛着障害	reactive attachment disorder（E）
反応(性)精神病	reactive psychosis（E）
反復	Iteration（D）
反復(性)うつ病性障害	recurrent depressive disorder（ICD-10）（E）
反復(性)過眠症	recurrent hypersomnia（E）
反復(性)強迫	repetition-compulsion（E），Wiederholungszwang（D）
半眠思考	Halbschlafdenken（D）
半盲*	hemianopsia（E）

ひ

悲哀の仕事，喪の仕事	mourning work（E），Trauerarbeit（D），travail de deuil（F）
被暗示性	suggestibility（E）
P-Fスタディ	Rosenzweig Picture-Frustration Study（E）
被影響感	sentiment d'influence（F）
被影響症候群	syndrome d'influence（A. Ceillier）（F）
被影響性	Beeinflußbarkeit（D）
被影響妄想	delusion of being influenced, delusion of control（E），Beeinflussungswahn（D）
被害妄想，迫害妄想，追跡妄想（解説用語）	delusion of persecution（E），Verfolgungswahn（D），délire de persécution（F）
比較精神医学	comparative psychiatry（E）
比較文化精神医学	transcultural psychiatry（E）
光過敏てんかん	photosensitive epilepsy（E）
光照射療法→高照度光療法	
ひきこもり	withdrawal（E）
非器質性睡眠障害	non organic sleep disorder（ICD-10）（E）
被虐性愛，マゾヒズム	masochism（E）
被虐待児症候群	battered-child syndrome（E）
備給	Besetzung（D），cathexis（E）
ピクノレプシー	pyknolepsy（E）
非言語的コミュニケーション	non-verbal communication（E）
非現実感	sentiment d'irréel（F）
非現実思考	dereistisches Denken（E. Bleuler）（D）
非行	delinquency（E）
被後見	Entmündigung（D），interdiction（E）
微細脳機能不全	minimal brain dysfunction（MBD）（E）
皮質下失語（症）	subcortical aphasia（E）
皮質下認知［痴呆］症	subcortical dementia（E）
皮質（性）失語（症）	cortical aphasia（E）

皮質盲	cortical blindness（E）, Rindenblindheit（D）
皮質聾	cortical deafness（E）
非社会（性）パーソナリティ［人格］障害	asocial personality disorder（ICD-9）, dissocial personality disorder（ICD-10）（E）
微小妄想	delusion of belittlement（E）, Kleinheitswahn（D）
ヒステリー	hysteria（E）
ヒステリー球	globus hystericus（L）
ヒステリー弓	hysterischer Bogen（D）
ヒステリー性格	hysterical character（E）
ヒステリー（性）精神病	hysterical psychosis（E）
ヒステリー（性）パーソナリティ［人格］障害	hysterical personality disorder（ICD-9）（E）
ヒステロエピレプシー（歴史用語）	hystéro-épilepsie（F）, hysteroepilepsy（E）
ひそめ眉	Gesichtsschneiden（D）
ピックウィック症候群	Pickwickian syndrome（E）
ピック病	Pick disease（E）
引越しうつ病	Umzugsdepression（J. Lange）（D）
必須症状	obligatory symptom（E）
筆跡学	graphology（E）
非定型自閉症	atypical autism（ICD-10, DSM-IV）（E）
非定型精神病	atypische Psychose（D）
否定妄想	Verneinungswahn（D）, délire de négation（F）
被動性*	passivité（F）
被毒妄想	Vergiftungswahn（D）
人見知り	stranger reaction, stranger anxiety（E）
一人歩き	free walking, unaided walking（E）
一人立ち	stand alone（E）
一人っ子	only child（E）

非24時間睡眠覚醒症候群	non-24-hour sleep-wake syndrome（E）
否認，否定	denial, negation（E），Verleugnung, Verneinung（D）
ひねくれ	Verschrobenheit（D）
皮膚寄生虫妄想	Dermatozoenwahn（K. A. Ekbom）（D）
ヒプスアリスミア	hypsarythmia（E）
ヒペルパチー*	hyperpathia（E），Hyperpathie（D）
ヒポコンドリー（性）基調	hypochondriacal temperament（森田正馬）（E）
被保佐，準禁治産	quasi-incompetence（E）
びまん性レビー小体病	diffuse Lewy body disease（DLBD）（E）
憑依	possession（E），Besessenheit（D）
憑依妄想，つきもの妄想	delusion of possession（E），Besessenheitswahn（D）
病院精神医学	hospital psychiatry（E），Anstaltspsychiatrie, Krankenhauspsychiatrie（D）
病感	Krankheitsgefühl（D）
表現型	phenotype（E）
表現失語（症）	expressive aphasia（E）
病識	insight into disease（E），Krankheitseinsicht（D）
表出性言語障害	expressive language disorder（ICD-10，DSM-III-R）（E）
病跡学	pathography（E），Pathographie（D）
病前性格	premorbid personality（E）
病相	phase（E），Phase（D）
病像形成的	pathoplastisch（K. Birnbaum）（D）
病像成因的	pathogenetisch（K. Birnbaum）（D）
病相頻発型気分障害⇒ラピッド・サイクラー	mood disorder with rapid cycling（DSM-IV）（E）
病態失認	anosognosia（E）
病的愛他主義	altruisme morbide（F）
病的欺瞞者	pathologischer Schwindler（D）

病的虚言	pathological lying（E）
病的合理主義	rationalisme morbide（E. Minkowski）（F）
病的賭博	pathological gambling（E）
病的酩酊	pathologischer Rausch（D）
病棟開放制	open door system（E）
病棟閉鎖制	closed door system（E）
非流暢失語（症）	nonfluent aphasia（E）
広場恐怖（症），アゴラフォビア	agoraphobia（E）
広場不安	Platzangst（D）
敏感関係妄想	sensitiver Beziehungswahn（E. Kretschmer）（D）
敏感パラノイア	Sensitivparanoia（D）
貧困妄想	delusion of poverty（E），Verarmungswahn（D）
ビンスワンガー病	Binswanger disease（E）
頻繁手術症，ポリサージェリ	polysurgery（E）

ふ

ファール病*	Fahr disease（E）
不安・恍惚精神病	Angst-Glückspsychose（K. Leonhard）（D）
不安障害	anxiety disorder（ICD-10, DSM-III）（E）
不安神経症	Angstneurose（D），anxiety neurosis（E）
不安定性人格→情動不安定（性）パーソナリティ［人格］障害	
不安ヒステリー	Angsthysterie（S. Freud）（D）
フィリアルセラピー	filial therapy（E）
風景構成法	landscape montage technique（E）
夫婦の分裂	marital schism（T. Lidz）（E）
夫婦のゆがみ	marital skew（T. Lidz）（E）
フェティシズム	fetishism（E）
フェニルケトン尿症*	phenylketonuria（E）

フェニル焦性ぶどう酸精神薄弱（歴史用語）	oligophrenia phenylpyruvica（L）
フェラグートの皺襞	Veraguthsche Falte（D），Veraguth fold（E）
フォーカシング	focusing（E）
負荷	Belastung（D）
不快気分	dysphoria（E）
賦活睡眠	activated sleep（E）
不感症→冷感症	
不機嫌	Verstimmtheit（D）
不機嫌躁病	dysphoric mania（E）
不器用な子ども症候群	clumsy child syndrome（E）
フーグ→遁走	
複合幻覚	complex hallucination（E）
複合性すね	komplizierte Schmollen（D）
複雑チック	complex tic（E）
複雑部分発作	complex partial seizure（E）
複雑酩酊	komplizierter Rausch（D）
複視*	diplopia（E），Doppelsehen（D）
複式簿記⇒二重見当識	doppelte Buchführung（E. Bleuler）（D）
副次妄想	Nebenwahn（D）
復讐性夜尿	revenge enuresis（E）
副腎白質ジストロフィー*	adrenoleukodystrophy（ALD）（E）
服装倒錯	transvestism（E）
腹皮反射*	abdominal skin reflex（E）
腹部てんかん	abdominal epilepsy（E）
腹壁深部反射*	abdominal deep reflex（E）
服薬遵守→コンプライアンス	
服薬不履行→ノンコンプライアンス	
不潔恐怖（症）	mysophobia（E）
ふざけ症	Witzelsucht（D）
不思議の国のアリス症候群	Alice-in-wonderland syndrome（E）
不死妄想	délire d'éternité（F）
不随意運動*	involuntary movement（E）

不全感	feeling of insufficiency（E）
ふたご研究	twin study（E），Zwillingsforschung（D）
二人組精神病	folie à deux（F）
不注意	inattention（E）
復権妄想（症，病）	délire de revendication（F）
物体失認	object agnosia（E）
物理的侵害妄想	physikalischer Beeinträchtigungswahn（D），delusion of injury with physical means（E）
不定時てんかん	diffuse Epilepsie（D. Janz）（D）
不適応	maladjustment（E）
不適応反応	maladjustment reaction（ICD-9）（E）
不適当人格	inadequate personality（E）
不統一狂気（歴史用語）	folie discordante（P. Chaslin）（F）
舞踏運動*	choreic movement（E）
不登校	non-attendance at school, severeness of school attendance（E）
舞踏病*	chorea（E）
舞踏アテトーゼ（運動）*	choreoathetosis（E）
浮動不安	free-floating anxiety（E）
ふとり型	pyknic（E），Pykniker（D）
不能症→性的不能症	
部分健忘	partial amnesia（E）
部分性愛	partialism（E）
部分対象関係	partial object relationship（E）
部分てんかん	partial epilepsy（E）
部分入院	partial hospitalization（E）
部分発作	partial seizure（E）
普遍的無意識　集合的無意識	collective unconscious（E），kollektives Unbewußtes（C. G. Jung）（D）
不眠	insomnia（E）
扶養義務者	person responsible for support（E）
プライマリーケア	primary care（E）
プライミング	priming（E）

プラセボ，偽薬	placebo（E）
プラダー-ウィリ症候群*	Prader-Willi syndrome（E）
ブラックアウト	black out（E）
フラッシュバック現象	flashback phenomenon（E），Nachhallphänomen（D）
フラッディング	flooding（E）
ブリケ症候群	Briquet syndrome（E）
不良行為	delinquent behavior（E）
プレコ（ッ）クス感	Praecoxgefühl（H. C. Rümke）（D）
フレゴリ症候群	Frégoli syndrome（E）
プレスビオフレニー	Presbyophrenie（D），presbyophrenia（E）
ブローカ失語（症）	Broca aphasia（E）
分画性能動催眠	fraktionierte Aktivhypnose（E. Kretschmer）（D）
文化結合症候群	culture-bound syndrome（E）
文化ショック，カルチャーショック	culture shock（E）
文化精神医学	cultural psychiatry（E）
文章完成テスト	sentence completion test（SCT）（E）
分節（性）失行	segmental apraxia（E）
憤怒けいれん	breath-holding spell，respiratory affect spasm（E）
分別もうろう状態	besonnener Dämmerzustand（D）
糞便愛	coprophilia（E）
分離個体化	separation-individuation（E）
分離不安	separation anxiety（E）
分離不安障害	separation anxiety disorder（E）
分裂病→統合失調症	

へ

平衡覚幻覚	hallucination of equilibrium（E）
閉眼失行（症）*	Lidschlußapraxie（D）
閉所恐怖（症）	claustrophobia（E）
併存（症）→コモビディティ	
ベビーブルー	baby blue（E）

ヘラー症候群	Heller syndrome（E）
ペラグラ精神病	pellagra psychosis（E）
辺縁症状	Randsymptom（D）
辺縁神経症	Randneurose（J. H. Schultz）（D）
変換運動障害*	adiadochokinesis, dysdiadochokinesis（E）
変形過多，変態過多	hypermetamorphosis（E）
変形視	metamorphopsia（E）
偏向発作	versive seizure（E）
変質（歴史用語）	dégénérescence（B. A. Morel）（F），degeneration（E），Entartung（D），
変質精神病	Degenerationspsychose（K. Kleist）（D）
偏執狂（歴史用語）	Verrücktheit（D）
弁証法的行動療法	dialectical behavioral therapy（E）
偏食	fastidium（E）
変身妄想	metamorphotischer Wahn（D）
片頭痛*	migrane（E）
変像（症）→パレイドリア	
片側頭痛*	hemicrania（E）
片側バリズム*	hemiballism（E）
ベンダー・ゲシュタルトテスト	Bender Gestalt Test（E）
ベントン視覚記銘検査	Benton visual retention test（E）
片麻痺*	hemiplegia（E）

ほ

保安処分	measures taken for the preservation of public security（E），Sicherungsmaßnahme（D）
哺育障害	feeding disorder（E）
防衛機制	Abwehrmechanismus（D），defense mechanism（E）
崩壊性行動障害	disruptive behavior disorders（DSM-Ⅲ-R）（E）
放火癖［症］	pyromania（E）
報酬系	reward system（E）

紡錘波	spindle（E）
砲弾ショック	shell shock（E）
放置恐怖（症）	paralipophobia（E）
包被法	zudeckende Methode（D）
補完医療	complementary medicine（E）
ボクサー脳症*	punch-drunk syndrome，boxer encephalopathy（E）
歩行障害*	gait disturbance（E）
歩行（性）自動症→徘徊自動症	
保護観察	probationary supervision（E）
保護作業場	sheltered workshop（E）
保護者	person responsible for protection（E）
保佐	curate（E）
保持，把持	retention（E）
ポジトロン断層撮影（法）	positron emission tomography（PET）（E）
補助自我	auxiliary ego（E）
ホスピス	hospice（E）
ホスピタリズム	hospitalism（E）
母性的養育	mothering（E）
母性遮断　母性剥奪	maternal deprivation（E）
保続	perseveration（E）
勃起障害	erectile disorder（ED）（E）
発作	seizure（E），Anfall（D），attaque，crise（F）
発作間欠期不機嫌症候群	inter-ictal dysphoric syndrome（E）
発作間欠期精神病	inter-ictal psychosis（E）
発作後精神病	postictal psychosis（E）
発作性，発作時	ictal（E）
発作（性）昏迷	ictal stupor（E）
発作後自動症	postictal automatism（E）
発作（性）自動症	ictal automatism（E）
発作発射	seizure discharge（E）
発端者	proband（E）
ポリグラフ	polygraph（E）

ポリグラフィ	polygraphy（E）
ポリサージェリ→頻繁手術症	
ポリソムノグラフィ	polysomnography（E）
ホールディング	holding（E）
本態性振戦*	essential tremor（E）
本能	instinct（E）

ま

埋葬恐怖（症）	taphephobia（E）
マイナーアノマリー，小形態異常	minor anomaly（E）
魔術的思考→呪術思考	
麻酔分析	narcoanalysis（E）
麻酔療法	narcotherapy（E）
マスターベーション，自慰	masturbation（E）
貧しい自閉	autisme pauvre（E. Minkowski）（F）
マゾヒズム→被虐性愛	
マタニティブルーズ	maternity blues（E）
まだら認知［痴呆］症	lacunar dementia（E）
的はずし応答，当意即答	approximate answer（E），Vorbeireden（D）
的はずし行動	Vorbeihandeln（D）
マニー親和型（性格）	typus manicus（D. v. Zerssen）（L）
麻痺（性）痴呆（歴史用語）	dementia paralytica（L）
麻痺（性）発作	paralytic attack（E）
幻の同居人	phantom boarder（E）
麻薬中毒	narcotics intoxication（E）
麻薬中毒者匿名会	narcotics anonymous（NA）（E）
マラリア療法	Malariakur（D）
マルキァファーヴァ-ビニャーミ病*	Marchiafava-Bignami disease（E）
慢性うつ病	chronic depression（E）
慢性幻覚精神病	psychose hallucinatoire chronique（G. Ballet）（F）
慢性幻触症	chronic tactile hallucination（E）
慢性自殺	chronic suicide（K. Menninger）（E）
慢性硬膜下血腫*	chronic subdural hematoma（E）

慢性疼痛	chronic pain（E）
慢性疲労症候群	chronic fatigue syndrome（E）
慢性躁病	chronic mania（E）
慢性妄想病	délire chronique（F）
マンダラ，曼荼羅	mandala（E）

み

ミオクローヌス*	myoclonus（E）
ミオクローヌスてんかん	myoclonus epilepsy（E）
ミオクロニー発作	myoclonic seizure（E）
味覚発作	gustatory seizure（E）
未完成婚	unconsummated marriage（E）
未視感	jamais vu（F）
身調べ	examining oneself（E）
水中毒	water intoxication（E）
見捨てられ抑うつ	abandonment depression（J. F. Masterson）（E）
ミスマッチ陰性電位	mismatch negativity（E）
道順障害	defective route finding（E）
満ち足りた無関心	belle indifférence（F）
ミトコンドリア脳筋症*	mitochondrial encephalomyopathy（E）
水俣病	Minamata disease（E）
ミネソタ多面人格目録	Minnesota Multiphasic Personality Inventory（MMPI）（E）
身ぶり自動症	gestural automatism（E）
三宅式記銘力テスト	Miyake recent memory scale（E），Merkprüfung（三宅鑛一）（D）
ミュンヒハウゼン症候群	Munchausen syndrome（E），Münchhausen Syndrom（D）
民事収容	civil commitment（E）
民族精神医学	ethnopsychiatry（E）

む

無為	abulia（E），Abulie（D）
無意識の	unconscious（E），unbewußt（D）

無縁体験	Fremdheitserlebnis（D）
無感情	apathy（E），Apathie（D）
無嗅覚	anosmia（E）
夢幻症	onirisme（E. Régis）（F）
夢幻精神病	oneirophrenia（L. J. Meduna）（E）
夢幻様状態	oneiroider Zustand（D），état oniroïde（F）
夢幻様体験型	oneiroide Erlebnisform（W. Mayer-Gross）（D）
無言（症）→緘黙（症）	
無作為化臨床試験	randomized clinical trial（RCT）（E）
矛盾性運動*	kinésie paradoxale（F）
無食欲症	anorexia（E）
むずむず脚症候群→下肢静止不能症候群	
むちゃ食い，気晴らし食い	binge eating（E）
むちゃ食い障害	binge-eating disorder（E）
無動*	akinesia（E）
無動機症候群	amotivational syndrome（E）
無動発作	akinetic seizure（E）
無動無言症	akinetic mutism（H. Cairns）（E）
無表情	amimia（E）
夢遊症，夢中遊行症	sleep walking，somnambulism（E），Schlafwandeln（D）
夢様意識	traumhaftes Bewußtsein（D）
夢様状態	dreamy state（H. Jackson）（E）
無力型（精神病質者）	Asthenische（Psychopathen）（K. Schneider）（D）
無論理思考	alogisches Denken（D）

め

明識困難状態	Schwerbesinnlichkeit（D）
明識性	Besinnlichkeit（D）
明識不能状態	Unbesinnlichkeit（D）
メージュ症候群*	Meige syndrome（E）
名称強迫，命名強迫	onomatomania（E）

酩酊	drunkenness（E），Rausch（D）
命令自動	Befehlsautomatie（D）
目覚め現象	awakenings（E）
メタ心理学，メタサイコロジー	metapsychology（E）
滅裂思考→思考滅裂	
メディアコンプレクス	Medea complex（E）
メディカル精神医学→身体管理精神医学	
めまい感	dizziness（E）
メランコリー	melancholia（E），Melancholie（D），mélancholie（F）
メランコリー型特徴	melancholic features（DSM-IV）（E）
メランコリー親和型（性格）	typus melancholicus（H. Tellenbach）（L）
メランコリーの激越発作，憂うつ激昂（歴史用語）	raptus melancholicus（L）

も

妄覚	Trugwahrnehmung（D）
妄想	delusion（E），Wahn（D），délire（F）
妄想意識性	Wahnbewußtheit（D）
妄想型統合失調症	paranoid schizophrenia, schizophrenia paranoid type（E）
妄想観念	Wahnidee（D），idée délirante（F）
妄想気分	delusional mood, delusional atmosphere（E），Wahnstimmung（D）
妄想激発→急性錯乱	
妄想構築	Wahngebäude（D）
妄想症→パラノイア	
妄想状態	paranoid state（E）
妄想（性）パーソナリティ［人格］障害	paranoid personality disorder（ICD-9, DSM-III）（E）
妄想性精神病	delusional psychosis（E）
妄想性障害	delusional disorder（E）
妄想体系	Wahnsystem（D）

妄想知覚	delusional perception（E）, Wahnwahrnehmung（D）
妄想（性）痴呆（歴史用語）	dementia paranoides（L）
妄想着想	Wahneinfall（D）
妄想追想	Wahnerinnerung（D）
妄想的解釈	wahnhafte Deutung（D）
妄想性人物誤認症候群	delusional misidentification syndrome（E）
妄想・統合失調質態勢→パラノイド・スキゾイド態勢	
妄想内容	Wahninhalt（D）
妄想発展	Wahnentwicklung（D）
妄想反応	paranoid reaction（E）
妄想表象	Wahnvorstellung（D）
妄想様観念	wahnhafte Idee（D）
もうろう状態	twilight state（E）, Dämmerzustand（D）, état crépusculaire（F）
燃え上がり効果→キンドリング	
燃えつき	burn-out（E）
持ち越し効果	hang-over effect（E）
モデリング	modeling（E）
喪の作業→悲哀の仕事	
モノマニー	monomanie（E. Esquirol）（F）, monomania（E）
模倣自動	Nachahmungsautomatie（D）
モラル療法	moral therapy, moral treatment（E）, traitment moral（F）
モリア	moria（E）
森田療法	Morita therapy（E）
モルヒネ（依存）症	morphinism（E）

や

夜間遺尿（症），夜尿症	enuresis nocturna（L）, nocturnal enuresis（E）
夜間飲水症候群	nocturnal drinking syndrome（E）

夜間摂食症候群	nocturnal eating syndrome（E）
夜間せん妄	night delirium（E）
夜間てんかん	Nachtepilepsie（D）
夜間病院→ナイトホスピタル	
夜間ミオクローヌス	nocturnal myoclonus（E）
夜驚症	pavor nocturnus（L），night terrors（E）
薬剤誘発性錐体外路症状	drug-induced extrapyramidal symptoms（E）
薬剤誘発性精神障害	drug-induced mental disorder（E）
薬物依存（症）	drug dependence（ICD-9）（E）
薬物血中濃度	plasma concentration of drug，plasma level of drug（E）
薬物嗜癖	drug addiction（E）
薬物相互作用	drug interaction（E）
薬物中毒	drug intoxication（E）
薬物乱用	drug abuse（E）
薬物離脱症候群	drug withdrawal syndrome（E）
薬物療法	drug therapy，pharmacotherapy（E）
やせ型	leptosomatic（E）
やせ願望	pursuit of thinness（E）
矢田部-ギルフォード性格検査	Yatabe-Guilford personality inventory（E）
山あらしジレンマ	porcupine dilemma（E）
病への逃避→疾病への逃避	

ゆ

優位半球	dominant（cerebral）hemisphere（E）
優格観念→支配観念	
有機溶剤乱用	organic solvent abuse，glue sniffing（E）
有棘赤血球舞踏病	chorea-acanthocytosis（E）
遊戯療法	play therapy（E）
夕暮れ症候群　たそがれ症候群	sundowner syndrome，sundowning syndrome（E）

有形幻覚	formed hallucination（E）
優生学	eugenics（E）
有病率	prevalence（E）
誘発うつ病	provozierte Depression（J. Lange）（D）
豊かな自閉	autisme riche（E. Minkowski）（F）
指失認	finger agnosia（E）
指しゃぶり	thumb sucking，finger sucking（E）
弓なり緊張，後弓反張	opisthotonus（E）
夢不安障害	dream anxiety disorder（E）
ゆりもどし再発	Kipprezidiv（D）

よ

養護学校	school for the handicapped（E）
養護ホーム	nursing home（E）
幼児語	baby talk（E）
幼児・児童用絵画統覚テスト	children's apperception test（CAT）（E）
陽性・陰性症状評価尺度	Positive and Negative Syndrome Scale（PANSS）（E）
陽性症状	positive symptom（E）
要素幻覚	photoma，elementary hallucination（E）
要素的認知機能障害	cognitive impairments with non dementia（CIND）（E）
要素発作	elementary seizure（E）
幼稚症	puerilism（E）
幼年痴呆（歴史用語）	dementia infantilis（T. Heller）（L）
予期神経症	Erwartungsneurose（D）
予期悲嘆	anticipatory grief（E）
予期不安	anticipatory anxiety，expectation anxiety（E），Erwartungsangst（D）
抑圧	repression（E），Verdrängung（D），refoulement（F）
抑うつ	depression（E）
抑うつ型（精神病質者）	Depressive（Psychopathen）（K. Schneider）（D）

抑うつ気分	depressed mood（E）
抑うつ状態	depressive state（E）
抑うつ神経症	depressive neurosis（E）
抑うつ反応	depressive reaction（E）
抑制	suppression（E），Unterdrückung（D），répression（F）
抑制消失，抑制欠如，脱抑制	Enthemmung（D）
欲動	drive（E），Trieb（D），pulsion（F）
欲動行為	Triebhandlung（D）
欲求不満，フラストレーション	frustration（E）
予防精神医学	preventive psychiatry（E）

ら

らい恐怖（症）（歴史用語）	lepraphobia（E）
ライ症候群*	Reye syndrome（E）
来談者中心療法，クライエント中心療法	client-centered therapy（C. R. Rogers）（E）
ライフイベント	life event（E）
ライフサイクル	life cycle（E）
ライフステージ	life stage（E）
ラター	latah（E）
ラピッド・サイクラー，病相頻発型	rapid cycler（E）
ラビット症候群	rabbit syndrome（E）
ラポール	rapport（F）
乱雑言語症→早口言語症	
ランダウ-クレフナー症候群	Landau-Kleffner syndrome（E）
乱買癖	oniomania（E），Kaufsucht（D）
乱用	abuse（E），Mißbrauch（D）

り

リエゾン精神医学⇒コンサルテーション・リエゾン精神医学	liaison psychiatry（E）
力動精神医学	dynamic psychiatry（E）
利口ぶり阿呆，釣り合い阿呆（歴史用語）	Verhältnisblödsinn（D），démence relative（F）

離人・現実感喪失症候群	depersonalization-derealization syndrome（E）
離人症	depersonalization（E）
離人症性障害	depersonalization disorder（DSM-III）（E）
リストカット，手首自傷	wrist-cutting（E）
理性的狂気（歴史用語）	folie raisonnante（F）
理想化	idealization（E）
離脱，退薬	withdrawal（E），Entziehung（D）
離脱，脱愛着	detachment（E）
離断症候群→大脳半球離断症候群	
立体感覚失認	astereognosia（E）
律動異常片頭痛*	dysrhythmic migrane（E）
律動性運動障害	rhythmic movement disorder（E）
リハビリテーション，社会復帰	rehabilitaiton（E）
リビド	libido（E）
罹病危険率	morbidity risk（E）
リビングウィル，生前遺書	living will（E）
リフレーミング	reframing（E）
リープマン現象	Liepmann phenomenon（E）
リペマニー（歴史用語）	lypémanie（E. Esquirol）（F）
流暢失語（症）	fluent aphasia（E）
瘤波	hump（E）
了解関連	verständlicher Zusammenhang（D）
了解心理学	verstehende Psychologie（D）
両価傾向	ambitendence（E）
両価性，アンビバレンツ	ambivalence（E），Ambivalenz（D）
領識	comprehension（E）
両性傾向，両性愛	bisexuality（E）
両性役割服装倒錯症	dual-role transvestism（E）
履歴現象	hysteresis（E）
臨死体験	near(-)death experience（E）
臨死患者	dying patient（E）
臨床心理学	clinical psychology（E）
臨床心理士	clinical psychologist（E）

る

類てんかん性格（歴史用語）	epileptoid personality（E）
類統合失調症，スキゾマニー	schizomanie（H. Claude）（F）
類破瓜病	Heboidophrenie（L. Kahlbaum）（D）
ループス精神病	lupus psychosis（E）

れ

例外状態	Ausnahmezustand（D）
冷感症	frigidity（E），Geschlechtskälte（D）
レクリエーション療法	recreational therapy（E）
レズビアン	lesbian（E）
劣位半球	subordinate（cerebral）hemisphere, nondominant hemisphere, recessive（nondoninant）cerebral hemisphere（E）
レッシュ-ナイハン症候群*	Lesch-Nyhan syndrome（E）
劣等感	feeling of inferiority（E），Minderwertigkeitsgefühl（D）
レット症候群（障害）	Rett syndrome（disorder）（E）
レビー小体型認知［痴呆］症	dementia with Lewy bodies（DLB）（E）
レム睡眠	REM（rapid eye movement）sleep（E）
レム潜時	REM latency（E）
レム睡眠行動障害	REM sleep behavior disorder（E）
恋愛妄想（病），被愛妄想（解説用語）	erotomania（E），Liebeswahn（D），érotomanie（G. G. de Clérambault）（F）
連結離断症候群→大脳半球離断症候群	
連合運動*	associated movement（E）
連合弛緩	loosening of association（E），Assoziationslockerung（D）
連続飲酒発作	drinking bout（E）
レンノックス-ガストー症候群	Lennox-Gastaut syndrome（E）
漣波	ripple wave（E）

ろ

蠟屈症	flexibilitas cerea (L), waxy flexibility (E)
老人虐待	elder abuse (E)
老人性愛	gerontophilia (E)
老人保健施設	elderly health care facility (E)
老人保健法	Health and Medical Service Law for the Aged (E)
老人ホーム	nursing home for the aged (E)
老年性記憶減退	age-associated memory impairment (AAMI) (E)
老年精神医学	geriatric psychiatry (E), Alterspsychiatrie (D)
老年精神病	senile psychosis (E)
老年認知[痴呆]症	senile dementia (E)
老年良性もの忘れ	benign (type of) senescent forgetfulness (E)
浪費癖	Verschwendungssucht (D)
弄糞，弄便	coprolagnia (E)
ロボトミー	lobotomy (E)
ロールシャッハテスト	Rorschach test (E)
ローレンス-ムーン-ビードル症候群	Laurence-Moon-Biedl syndrome (E)
ロゴテラピー	Logotherapie (V. E. Frankl) (D)
露出症	exhibitionism (E)
論理療法	rational emotive therapy (E)

わ

矮小脳症*	micr[o]encephaly[-lia] (E)
わが道を行く行動	going my way behavior (E)
ワーキングメモリー→作動[働]記憶	
わざとらしさ，衒奇症	mannerism (E), Manieriertheit (D)
笑い発作	Lachschlag (D)
湾岸戦争症候群	Gulf-War syndrome (E)
ワーンジン，妄想錯乱（歴史用語）（解説用語）	Wahnsinn (D)

外 国 語 索 引

abandonment depression（J. F. Masterson）（E）	97
abasia（E）	43
abdominal deep reflex（E）	91
abdominal epilepsy（E）	91
abdominal skin reflex（E）	91
Abhängigkeit（D）	5
Ablenkbarkeit（D）	75
abnormal drunkenness（E）	5
abnorme Körpersensation（D）	5
abnorme Persönlichkeit（D）	51
abnormer Rausch（D）	5
abreaction（E）	11
absence（F）	27
absolute bedrest（Morita therapy）（E）	63
Abstammungswahn（D）	27
Abstinenzerscheinung（D）	24
Abstinenzsymptom（D）	24
abstract attitude（E）	72
abstraktes Verhalten（K. Goldstein）（D）	72
abulia（E）	97
Abulie（D）	97
abuse（E）	20, 103
Abwehrmechanismus（D）	94
acalculia（E）	42
acataphasia（E）	28
acathisia（E）	57
acceptance（E）	47
accessibility（E）	66
accident neurosis（E）	35
accident proneness（E）	40
accommodation reflex（E）	73
Achsensymptom（D）	72

A

acrophobia (E)	31
acting out (E)	32
action tremor (E)	76
activated sleep (E)	91
Act on Medical Care and Treatment for Persons who have caused serious Cases under the Condition of Insanity (E)	54
acute alcohol intoxication (E)	21
acute and transient psychotic disorder (ICD-10) (E)	21
acute brain syndrome (E)	21
acute cannabinoid intoxication (E)	21
acute cocaine intoxication (E)	21
acute confusional state (E)	21
acute disseminated encephalomyelitis (ADEM) (E)	21
acute dystonia (E)	21
acute hallucinogen intoxication (E)	21
acute intoxication (E)	21
acute nicotine intoxication (E)	21
acute opioid intoxication (E)	21
acute polymorphic psychotic disorder (E)	21
acute schizophrenia-like psychotic disorder (E)	21
acute stress disorder (DSM-IV-TR) (E)	21
acute stress reaction (ICD-10) (E)	21
addiction (E)	44
adherence (E)	1
adiadochokinesis (E)	94
adjustment disorder (ICD-10, DSM-III) (E)	74
admission for medical care and protection (E)	6
admission with social reasons (E)	44
adolescence (E)	62
adolescent paranoia (E)	40
adolescent psychiatry (E)	62
adrenoleukodystrophy (ALD) (E)	91
adult children (E)	1
adult guardianship (E)	62

adult guardian system (E)	62
advanced sleep phase (E)	56
adversive seizure (E)	32
advocacy (E)	29
advocacy for community welfare (E)	70
aerophagia (E)	25
affect (E)	48
affect (F)	48
affective disorder (ICD-10) (E)	15
affective illness (E)	16
Affekt (D)	48
Affektinkontinenz (D)	49
Affektivität (D)	49
Affektlabilität (D)	49
Affektpsychose (D)	15
Affektstupor (D)	48
Affekttonusverlust (D)	49
aftercare (E)	1
age-associated memory impairment (AAMI) (E)	106
aged society (E)	73
agenesis of corpus callosum (E)	83
aggression (E)	30
agitierte Depression (D)	26
agnosia (E)	42
agnosie d'utilisation (J. Morlaas) (F)	48
agonist (E)	1
agoraphobia (E)	90
agrammatism (E)	43
agraphia (E)	42
agressologie (F)	53
agressology (E)	53
aichmophobia (E)	64
AIDS dementia complex (E)	8
aid system for employer (岡上和雄) (E)	50

Ajase complex（古澤平作）（E）	1
akathisia（E）	57
akinesia（E）	98
akinetic mutism（H. Cairns）（E）	98
akinetic seizure（E）	98
Aktivitätsbewußtsein（D）	82
Aktivitätsmangel（D）	82
Aktualneurose（S. Freud）（D）	28
alcohol（E）	2
alcohol abuse（E）	2
alcohol dependence（E）	2
alcohol epilepsy（E）	2
alcoholic hallucinosis（E）	2
alcoholic intolerance（E）	2
alcoholic psychosis（E）	2
alcoholics anonymous（AA）（E）	2
alcoholic withdrawal delirium（E）	2
alcohol-induced（DSM-IV）（E）	2
alcohol-induced anxiety disorders（E）	3
alcohol-induced disorders（E）	3
alcohol-induced mood disorders（E）	2
alcohol-induced persisting amnestic disorders（E）	2
alcohol-induced persisting dementia（E）	3
alcohol-induced psychotic disorders（E）	3
alcohol-induced sexual dysfunction（E）	3
alcohol-induced sleep disorders（E）	3
alcohol intoxication（E）	2
alcohol intoxication delirium（E）	2
alcoholism（E）	2
alcohol-related disorders（E）	2
alcohol test（E）	6
alcohol use disorders（E）	2
alcohol withdrawal（E）	2
alexia（E）	42

alexia without agraphia (E)	47
alexithymia (E)	42
Alexithymie (D)	42
algolagnia (E)	2, 77
algomania (E)	77
algophobia (E)	77
algorism (E)	2
Alice-in-wonderland syndrome (E)	91
Alkoholismus (D)	2
Alkoholtrinkversuch (D)	6
allgemeine Amnesie (D)	64
Allmachtsgefühl (D)	65
allochiria (E)	3
allomnesia (E)	33
Allopsyche (C. Wernicke) (D)	10
alogisches Denken (D)	98
alopecanthropia (E)	19
alpha coma (E)	3
alpha wave (E)	3
alternating consciousness (E)	32
alternating personality (E)	32
alternierende Persönlichkeit (D)	32
alternierendes Bewußtsein (D)	32
Alterspsychiatrie (D)	106
altruisme morbide (F)	89
Alzheimer disease (E)	3
amaxophobia (E)	83
ambitendence (E)	104
ambivalence (E)	104
Ambivalenz (D)	104
ambulatory automatism (E)	83
Amentia (D)	2
amimia (E)	98
ammon horn sclerosis (E)	4

amnesia (E) ... 29
amnesia of personal history (E) ... 64
amnésie élective (F) ... 64
amnes(t)ic aphasia (E) ... 29
amnes(t)ic syndrome (E) ... 29
amok (E) ... 2
Amok (D) ... 2
amotivational syndrome (E) ... 76, 98
amphetamine (E) ... 3
amphetamine abuse (E) ... 3
amphetamine dependence (E) ... 3
amphetamine-induced (DSM-IV) (E) ... 3
amphetamine-induced disorders (E) ... 4
amphetamine-induced mood disorders (E) ... 4
amphetamine-induced psychotic disorders (E) ... 4
amphetamine-induced sexual dysfunction (E) ... 4
amphetamine-induced sleep disorders (E) ... 4
amphetamine intoxication (E) ... 3
amphetamine intoxication delirium (E) ... 3
amphetamine psychosis (E) ... 12
amphetamine-related disorders (E) ... 3
amphetamine use disorders (E) ... 3
amphetamine withdrawal (E) ... 3
amusia (E) ... 42
anaclitic (E) ... 5
anaclitic depression (R. Spitz) (E) ... 5
anal character (E) ... 32
anality (E) ... 32
anal phase [stage] (E) ... 32
anancastic neurosis (E) ... 62
anancastic personality disorder (E) ... 62
Anankast (D) ... 23
anarthria (E) ... 30, 42
anarthrie (F) ... 30

Anfall (D)	95
Angst-Glückspsychose (K. Leonhard) (D)	90
Angsthysterie (S. Freud) (D)	90
Angstneurose (D)	90
anhedonia (E)	11
animal magnetism (E)	77
anisocoria (E)	77
anniversary reaction (E)	19
anomic aphasia (E)	43
anorexia (E)	98
anorexia nervosa (L)	53
anosmia (E)	98
anosodiaphoria (E)	43
anosognosia (E)	89
Anstaltspsychiatrie (D)	89
antagonist (E)	3
anterograde amnesia (E)	63
anthropophobia (E)	67
antialcoholic agent (E)	29
antianxiety drug (E)	32
anticholinergic drug (E)	31
anticipatory anxiety (E)	102
anticipatory grief (E)	102
anticonvulsant (E)	30
antidepressant (E)	30
antiepileptic drug (E)	32
antiepileptics (E)	32
antipsychiatry (E)	86
antipsychotic drug (E)	31
antipsychotics (E)	31
antisocial personality disorder (DSM-III) (E)	86
Anton syndrome (E)	3
Antrieb (D)	85
Antriebsapraxie (D)	85

Antriebsmangel （D） ……………………………………………… 85
anxiety disorder （ICD-10，DSM-III）（E） ……………… 90
anxiety neurosis （E） …………………………………………… 90
anxiolytic drug （E） …………………………………………… 32
anxiolytics （E） ………………………………………………… 32
apallic syndrome （E） ………………………………………… 42
apallisches Syndrom （E. Kretschmer）（D） ……………… 42
Apathie （D） …………………………………………………… 98
apathy （E） ……………………………………………………… 98
aphasia （E） …………………………………………………… 42
Aphasie （D） …………………………………………………… 42
aphonia （E） …………………………………………………… 42
Aphonie （D） …………………………………………………… 42
apperception （E） ……………………………………………… 76
approximate answer （E） ……………………………………… 96
apractognosia （E） ……………………………………………… 42
apraxia （E） ……………………………………………………… 42
apraxia for dressing （E） ……………………………………… 71
apraxia of lid opening （E） …………………………………… 10
Apraxie （D） …………………………………………………… 42
Arbeitstherapie （D） …………………………………………… 36
archaic （E） ……………………………………………………… 65
archaisches Denken （D） ……………………………………… 67
Archetypus （C. G. Jung）（D） ……………………………… 28
argy[i]rophilic grain dementia （AGD）（E） ……………… 39
arithmetic disorder （ICD-10）（E） ………………………… 37
arithmomania （E） ……………………………………………… 26
arrested paresis （E） …………………………………………… 74
arrest seizure （E） ……………………………………………… 74
arriération mentale （F） ……………………………………… 60
Artikulationsstörung （D） …………………………………… 30
art therapy （E） ………………………………………………… 26
Asher syndrome （E） …………………………………………… 9
asocial personality disorder （ICD-9）（E） ………………… 88

asomatognosia (E)	54
Asperger syndrome (E)	1
aspontaneity (E)	44
associated movement (E)	105
Assoziationslockerung (D)	105
astasia (E)	43
astatic seizure (E)	43
astereognosia (E)	104
asterixis (E)	41
Asthenische (Psychopathen) (K. Schneider) (D)	98
astraphobia (E)	14
asymbolia (E)	42
asymbolia for pain (E)	74
ataxia (E)	8
ataxic gait (E)	42
athetosis (E)	1
athletic (E)	77
A-T split (E)	8
attaque (F)	95
attempt of suicide (E)	40
attention-deficit/hyperactivity disorder (ADHD) (DSM-IV) (E)	72
attention deficit disorder (ADD) (DSM-III) (E)	71
atypical autism (ICD-10, DSM-IV) (E)	88
atypische Psychose (D)	88
audible thoughts (E)	31
auditogenic seizure (E)	73
auditory agnosia (E)	73
auditory hallucination (E)	29
auditory hallucinatory seizure (E)	29
auditory seizure (E)	73
aufdeckende Methode (D)	50
Aufwachepilepsie (D. Janz) (D)	12
aura (E)	64
Auslegung (D)	10

Ausnahmezustand (D) 105
autism (E) 44
autisme pauvre (E. Minkowski) (F) 96
autisme riche (E. Minkowski) (F) 102
Autismus (D) 44
autistic disorder (E) 44
autistische Psychopathie (H. Asperger) (D) 44
autobiographic memory (E) 43
autochthones Denken (D) 41
autochthonous idea (E) 41
autoerotism (E) 41
autogenes Training (J. H. Schultz) (D) 51
autogenic training (E) 51
automatic thought (E) 43
automatic writing (E) 43
automatism (E) 43
automatisme ambulatoire (F) 83
automatisme mental (G. G. de Clérambault) (F) 59
automatisme psychologique (P. Janet) (F) 55
autonomic dystonia (E) 51
autonomic seizure (E) 51
Autopsyche (C. Wernicke) (D) 79
autoscopy (E) 40
Autoskopie (D) 40
autosuggestion (E) 39
autotopagnosia (E) 40
auxiliary ego (E) 95
avoidant personality disorder (DSM-III) (E) 11
awakening epilepsy (E) 12
awakenings (E) 99
axial amnesia (E) 39
axial symptom (E) 72
babbling (E) 79
baby blue (E) 93

baby talk (E) ··· 102
bacillophobia (E) ··· 35
Bálint syndrome (E) ··· 85
Balkenapraxie (D) ·· 83
Balkenmangel (D) ·· 83
ballism (E) ·· 85
basic fault (M. Balint) (E) ·· 19
basic symptom (E) ··· 20
basic trust (E. H. Erikson) (E) ··· 20
battered-child syndrome (E) ··· 87
battered parents syndrome (E) ·· 9
Baumtest (D) ·· 83
Beachtungswahn (D) ·· 72
Bedeutungswahn (D) ··· 6
Beeinflußbarkeit (D) ·· 87
Beeinflussungswahn (D) ·· 87
Beeinträchtigungwahn (D) ·· 51
Befehlsautomatie (D) ··· 99
Begnadigungswahn (D) ·· 45
Begriffszerfall (D) ·· 11
Beharrungsneigung (D) ·· 33
behavior (E) ·· 32
behavior therapy (E) ··· 32
Bekanntheitsgefühl (D) ·· 19
Bekehrung (D) ·· 11
Bekehrungserlebnis (D) ·· 11
Bekleidungsapraxie (D) ·· 71
Belastung (D) ·· 91
belle indifférence (F) ··· 97
Bender Gestalt Test (E) ··· 94
benign epilepsy of children with centro-temporal EEG foci (BECCT) (E) ········ 72
benign (type of) senescent forgetfulness (E) ·· 106
Benommenheit (D) ··· 35
Benton visual retention test (E) ·· 94

benumbness (E)	35
Beobachtungswahn (D)	72
bereavement (E)	44
Berührungshalluzination (D)	29
Berührungsillusion (D)	36
Beschäftigungsdelirium (D)	36
Beschäftigungsdrang (D)	36
Beschäftigungstherapie (D)	36
Besessenheit (D)	89
Besessenheitswahn (D)	89
Besetzung (D)	87
Besinnlichkeit (D)	98
besonnener Dämmerzustand (D)	93
Bestehlungswahn (D)	76
bestiality (E)	45
Bettsucht (D)	13
Bewegungsdrang (D)	8
Bewegungsstereotypie (D)	8
Bewegungssturm (D)	8
bewilderment (E)	35
Bewußtheit (D)	4
Bewußtlosigkeit (D)	5
Bewußtsein (D)	4
Bewußtseinseinengung (D)	4
Bewußtseinsinhalt (D)	5
Bewußtseinsschwelle (D)	4
Bewußtseinsstörung (D)	4
Bewußtseinstrübung (D)	4
Bewußtseinsveränderung (D)	5
Beziehungswahn (D)	15
Bildagglutination (D)	26
Bildhaftigkeit (D)	13
binge eating (E)	98
binge-eating disorder (E)	98

Binswanger disease (E)	90
bio-feedback therapy (E)	83
biological psychiatry (E)	62
bipolar affective disorder (ICD-10) (E)	15
bipolar affective disorder (E)	65
bipolar depression (E)	65
bipolar disorder (DSM-IV-TR) (E)	65
bipolar I disorder (DSM-IV-TR) (E)	65
bipolar II disorder (DSM-IV-TR) (E)	65
birth trauma (E)	46
bisexuality (E)	104
black out (E)	93
blaptophobia (E)	12
Blickanfall (D)	72
Blickkrampf (D)	72
Blitz-Nick-Salaam Krampf (B-N-S Krampf) (D)	75
blocking (E)	78
blocking of thought (E)	39
blood brain barrier (BBB) (E)	26
blunted affect (E)	16
body dysmorphic disorders (E)	54
body image (E)	54
body schema (E)	54
borderline case (E)	22
borderline intellectual functioning (DSM-IV) (E)	22
borderline personality disorder (DSM-III) (E)	22
borderline personality organization (O. Kernberg) (E)	22
bouffée délirante (F)	21
bovine spongiform encephalopathy (BSE) (E)	7
boxer encephalopathy (E)	95
bradykinesia (E)	8
bradylalia (E)	84
bradyphrenia (E)	58
brain concussion (E)	82

brain contusion (E)	82
brain death (E)	82
brainedness (E)	17
brain pathology (E)	82
brain wash (E)	65
breath-holding spell (E)	4, 93
breathing-related sleep disorder (E)	33
Brief Psychiatric Rating Scale (BPRS) (E)	14
brief psychotherapy (E)	14, 48
brief psychotic disorder (DSM-IV) (E)	70
brief reactive psychosis (DSM-III) (E)	70
bright light treatment (E)	31
Briquet syndrome (E)	93
Broca aphasia (E)	93
buccofacial apraxia (E)	32
buffoonery syndrome (E)	76
bulbar palsy (E)	21
bulbar paralysis (E)	21
bulimia (E)	13, 67
bulimia nervosa (L)	53
burn-out (E)	100
ça (F)	9
caffeine-induced anxiety disorder (E)	14
caffeine-induced sleep disorder (E)	14
caffeine intoxication (E)	14
callosal agenesis (E)	83
cannabis (E)	68
cannabis abuse (E)	68
cannabis dependence (E)	68
cannabis-induced disorders (E)	68
cannabis intoxication (E)	68
cannabis intoxication delirium (E)	68
cannabis-related disorders (E)	68
Capgras syndrome (E)	14

carcinophobia (E)	15
cardiac neurosis (E)	54
care manager (E)	26
case management (E)	26
caseness (E)	51
castration anxiety (E)	24
catalepsy (E)	13
cataplexy (E)	69
catatonia (E)	24
categorical attitude (E)	86
catharsis (E)	13
cathexis (E)	87
causalgia (E)	45
cénesthésie (F)	67
cenesthopathy (E)	67
cénestopathie (F)	67
central pontine myelinolysis (E)	22
centrencephalic seizure (E)	72
cerebral arteriosclerosis (E)	82
cerebral dominance (E)	68
cerebral edema (E)	82
cerebral hemisphere disconnection [disconnexion] syndrome (E)	68
cerebral lateralization (E)	68
cerebral palsy (E)	82
cerebral syphilis (E)	82
certification for health and welfare of the person with mental disorder (E)	60
character neurosis (E)	56
characterology (E)	56
Charakterveränderung (D)	56
Charles Bonnet syndrome (E)	45
checking compulsion (E)	12
chief complaint (E)	46
child abuse (E)	43
child and adolescent antisocial behavior (E)	49

child guidance center（E） ... 43
childhood absence epilepsy（E） ... 49
childhood depression（E） ... 49
childhood disintegrative disorder（DSM-IV）（E） ... 49
childhood neurosis（E） ... 43
childhood schizophrenia（E） ... 43
child psychiatry（E） ... 43
children's apperception test（CAT）（E） ... 102
Child Welfare Law（E） ... 43
choked disc（E） ... 7
cholinesterase inhibitor（E） ... 34
chorea（E） ... 92
chorea-acanthocytosis（E） ... 101
chorea minor（E） ... 49
choreic movement（E） ... 92
choreoathetosis（E） ... 92
chronic depression（E） ... 96
chronic fatigue syndrome（E） ... 97
chronic mania（E） ... 97
chronic pain（E） ... 97
chronic subdural hematoma（E） ... 96
chronic suicide（K. Menninger）（E） ... 96
chronic tactile hallucination（E） ... 96
chronobiology（E） ... 38
chronological age（E） ... 57
chronopsychiatry（E） ... 38
chronotherapy（E） ... 38
cingulate seizure（E） ... 67
circadian rhythm（E） ... 11
circadian rhythm sleep disorder（E） ... 11
circumstantiality（E） ... 7
civil commitment（E） ... 97
clasp-knife phenomenon（E） ... 10
claustrophobia（E） ... 93

clavus (L)	25
cleptomania (E)	77
cleptophobia (E)	63
client-centered therapy (C. R. Rogers) (E)	103
clinical guidance in way of life (E)	57
clinical psychologist (E)	104
clinical psychology (E)	104
clinomania (E)	13
clonic convulsion (E)	16
clonus (E)	16
closed door system (E)	90
clouding of consciousness (E)	4
clownism (E)	9
clumsy child syndrome (E)	91
cluster headache (E)	25
cluttering (E)	85
cocaine (E)	33
cocaine abuse (E)	33
cocaine dependence (E)	33
cocaine-induced anxiety disorder (E)	33
cocaine-induced disorders (E)	33
cocaine-induced mood disorder (E)	33
cocaine-induced psychotic disorder (E)	33
cocaine-induced sexual dysfunction (E)	33
cocaine-induced sleep disorder (E)	33
cocaine intoxication (E)	33
cocaine intoxication delirium (E)	33
cocaine-related disorders (DSM-IV) (E)	33
cocaine use disorders (E)	33
cocaine withdrawal (E)	33
cocainism (E)	33
co-dependency (E)	21
coenästhetische Schizophrenie (G. Huber) (D)	67
cognitive deficit (E)	81

cognitive enhancer (E)	32
cognitive impairments with non dementia (CIND) (E)	102
cognitive psychology (E)	81
cognitive therapy (E)	81
cogwheel rigidity (E)	84
collectionism (E)	45
collectionnisme (F)	45
collective unconscious (E)	92
collectomania (E)	45
color anomia (E)	39
color-hearing (E)	38
coma (E)	35
coma vigil (F)	12
combined type (E)	72
co-medical (E)	34
communication disorder (E)	34
community life support center for the person with mental disorder (E)	60
community life support work for the person with mental disorder (E)	59
community organization (E)	70
community psychiatry (E)	70
comorbidity (E)	34
comparative psychiatry (E)	86
compartment model (E)	35
compensation neurosis (E)	83
complementary medicine (E)	95
complex (E)	35
complex hallucination (E)	91
complex partial seizure (E)	91
complex tic (E)	91
compliance (E, F)	35
comportement (F)	32
comprehension (E)	104
compromise formation (E)	68
compulsion (E)	23

compulsive act（E）	23
compulsive manipulation of tools（E）	76
compulsive personality disorder（DSM-III）（E）	23
computed tomography（E）	35
computerized tomography（CT）（E）	35
concentration camp syndrome（E）	22
concentric contraction of visual field（E）	20
condensation（E）	1
conditioned reflex（E）	48
conditioning（E）	48
conduct disorder（DSM-III）（E）	66
conduction aphasia（E）	75
conduct retardation（E）	30
confabulation（E）	36
confidentiality（E）	47
confinement at one's family home（E）	41
conflict（E）	14
confusion（E）	36
confusion mentale（F）	58
confusion mentale primitive（P. Chaslin）（F）	29
conjoint psychotherapy（E）	77
conjugate deviation of eyes（E）	23
conjugate gaze（E）	23
consciousness（E）	4
constructional agraphia（E）	31
constructional apraxia（E）	31
constructive agraphia（E）	31
constructive apraxia（E）	31
consultation-liaison psychiatry（E）	35
contact（E）	63
contact vital avec la réalité（E. Minkowski）（F）	29
contractual capacity（E）	30
contre-transfert（F）	20
conversion（E）	11, 75

conversion disorder（ICD-10，DSM-III）（E）	75
conversion experience（E）	11
conversion hysteria（E）	75
convulsion（E）	26
convulsive seizure（E）	26
convulsive therapy（E）	26
coordination（E）	22
coping（E）	34
coprolagnia（E）	106
coprolalia（E）	9
coprophagia（E）	50
coprophilia（E）	93
Cornelia de Lange syndrome（E）	34
Cornell Medical Index（CMI）（E）	34
corpus callosum syndrome（E）	83
cortical aphasia（E）	87
cortical blindness（E）	88
cortical deafness（E）	88
corticobasal degeneration（CBD）（E）	68
Cotard syndrome（E）	34
counseling（E）	12
counter-transference（E）	20
couvade syndrome（E）	24
crane phenomenon（E）	25
cretinism（E）	25
Creuzfeldt-Jakob disease（E）	25
criminal psychiatry（E）	86
criminal responsibility（E）	62
crise（F）	95
crise convulsive（F）	26
crisis intervention（E）	17
cryptomnesia（E）	64
cryptomnesie（T. Flournoy）（F）	64
cultural psychiatry（E）	93

culture-bound syndrome (E) ... 93
culture shock (E) ... 93
curate (E) ... 95
custodial care (E) ... 30
cyclic schizopherenia (E) ... 47
cyclic vomiting (E) ... 45
cycloid (E) ... 47
cyclothymia (E) ... 19
cyclothymia (ICD-10) (E) ... 47
cyclothymic disorder (E) ... 20
cynanthropy ** (E) ... 6
daily fluctuation (E) ... 80
daily living training stage (Morita therapy) (E) ... 45
Dämmerzustand (D) ... 100
Daseinsanalyse (D) ... 29
Dauerbad (D) ... 41
Dauerschlaf (D) ... 41
day care (E) ... 74
day dream (E) ... 84
day hospital (E) ... 74
decerebrate posture (E) ... 50
Deckerinnerung (S. Freud) (D) ... 7
declarative memory (E) ... 73
decorticate posture (E) ... 50
defective route finding (E) ... 97
defect state (E) ... 27
Defektzustand (D) ... 27
defense mechanism (E) ... 94
degeneration (E) ... 94
Degenerationspsychose (K. Kleist) (D) ... 94
dégénérescence (B. A. Morel) (F) ... 94
deinstitutionalization (E) ... 69
déjà éprouvé (F) ... 17
déjà vécu (F) ... 19

D

déjà vu (F)	18
delayed echolalia (E)	70
delayed sleep phase syndrome (E)	56
delinquency (E)	87
delinquent behavior (E)	93
délire (F)	99
délire aigu (F)	21
délire chronique (F)	97
délire de fabulation (F)	24
délire de grandeur (F)	34
délire de négation (F)	88
délire de persécution (F)	87
délire de préjudice (F)	51
délire de protection (F)	46
délire de relation (F)	15
délire de revendication (F)	92
délire d'éternité (F)	91
délire d'imagination (E. Dupré) (F)	25
délire d'interprétation (P. Sérieux & J. Capgras) (F)	10
delirium (E)	65
delirium tremens (L)	54
delusion (E)	99
delusional atmosphere (E)	99
delusional disorder (E)	99
delusional misidentification syndrome (E)	100
delusional mood (E)	99
delusional perception (E)	100
delusional psychosis (E)	99
delusion of amnesty (E)	45
delusion of being avoided (E)	19
delusion of being influenced (E)	87
delusion of belittlement (E)	88
delusion of control (E)	87
delusion of guilt (E)	35

delusion of injury (E)	51
delusion of injury with physical means (E)	92
delusion of invention (E)	85
delusion of jealousy (E)	42
delusion of observation (E)	72
delusion of persecution (E)	87
delusion of possession (E)	89
delusion of poverty (E)	90
delusion of reference (E)	15
delusion of robbery (E)	76
démence (F)	81
démence relative (F)	103
dementia (E)	80
dementia infantilis (T. Heller) (L)	102
dementia paralytica (L)	96
dementia paranoides (L)	100
dementia phantasitica (L)	25
dementia praecocissima (De Sanctis) (L)	35, 207
dementia praecox (E. Kraepelin) (L)	66
dementia simplex (L)	70
dementia with Lewy bodies (DLB) (E)	105
Demenz (D)	81
demonomania (E)	1
demyelinating disease (E)	69
denervation (E)	69
denial (E)	89
denial of illness (E)	43
Denkfaulheit (D)	14, 39
Denkhemmung (D)	39
Denksperrung (D)	39
Denkstörung (D)	39
dependence (E)	5
dependent (E)	5
dependent personality disorder (DSM-III) (E)	5

depersonalization（E） ········· 104
depersonalization-derealization syndrome（E） ········· 104
depersonalization disorder（DSM-III）（E） ········· 104
dépossession（F） ········· 40
depressed mood（E） ········· 103
depression（E） ········· 7, 102
Depression（D） ········· 7
dépression（F） ········· 7
Depressive（Psychopathen）（K. Schneider）（D） ········· 102
depressive disorders（E） ········· 8
depressive episode（E） ········· 7
depressive neurosis（E） ········· 103
depressive pseudodementia（E） ········· 8
depressive reaction（E） ········· 103
depressive state（E） ········· 103
depressive stupor（E） ········· 8
depth psychology（E） ········· 54
Derealisation（W. Mayer-Gross）（D） ········· 28
dereistisches Denken（E. Bleuler）（D） ········· 87
Dermatozoenwahn（K. A. Ekbom）（D） ········· 89
désagrégation psychique（F） ········· 58
descent delusion（E） ········· 27
descriptive psychiatry（E） ········· 19
desensitization therapy（E） ········· 69
designated hospital（E） ········· 43
designated physician of mental health（E） ········· 61
Desorientiertheit（D） ········· 42
detachment（E） ········· 104
detention for psychiatric evidence（E） ········· 16
deterioration（E） ········· 32
Deutung（D） ········· 10
developmental age（E） ········· 84
developmental alexia and agraphia（E） ········· 84
developmental aphasia（E） ········· 84

developmental ariculation disorder (DSM-III) (E) ········· 84
developmental coordination disorder (DSM-III-R) (E) ········· 84
developmental diagnosis (E) ········· 84
developmental disorder (E) ········· 84
developmental quotient (DQ) (E) ········· 84
developmental task (E) ········· 84
developmental test (E) ········· 84
diagnosis by exclusion (E) ········· 50
Diagnostic and Statistical Manual of Mental Disorders (DSM) (APA) (E) ····· 60
diagnostic criteria (E) ········· 55
diagnostic imaging (E) ········· 13
dialectical behavioral therapy (E) ········· 94
Diaschisis (C v. Monakow) (D) ········· 74
didactic analysis (E) ········· 21
diencephalic syndrome (E) ········· 16
diencephalosis (E) ········· 16
difficulty of falling asleep (E) ········· 80
diffuse Epilepsie (D. Janz) (D) ········· 92
diffuse Lewy body disease (DLBD) (E) ········· 89
diffuse neurofibrillary tangles with calcification (DNTC) (E) ········· 63
diminished responsibility (E) ········· 53
diplopia (E) ········· 91
dipsomania (E) ········· 14
disease (E) ········· 42
disease entity (E) ········· 42
disinhibited attachment disorder (E) ········· 69
disorder of written expression (E) ········· 50
disorganaized schizophrenia (E) ········· 11
disorientation (E) ········· 42
displacement (E) ········· 9
disruptive behavior disorders (DSM-III-R) (E) ········· 94
dissimulation (E) ········· 42
dissocial personality disorder (ICD-10) (E) ········· 88
dissociation (E, F) ········· 11

dissociative amnesia (E) ... 11
dissociative disorder (E) ... 11
dissociative fugue (E) ... 11
dissociative hysteria (E) ... 11
dissociative identity disorder (DSM-IV) (E) ... 11
dissolution (H. Jackson) (E) ... 11
distractibility (E) ... 75
distructive behavier disorder (E) ... 83
disturbance of consciousness (E) ... 4
disturbance of memorization (E) ... 20
disturbance of thought (E) ... 39
disturbance of visual attention (E) ... 37
diurnal enuresis (E) ... 72
diurnal fluctuation (E) ... 80
dizziness (E) ... 99
doll's eye phenomenon (reflex, test, sign) (E) ... 81
domestic violence (DV) (E) ... 14
dominant (cerebral) hemisphere (E) ... 101
dominierende Vorstellung (D) ... 44
Doppeldenken (D) ... 80
Doppelgänger (D) ... 80
Doppelsehen (D) ... 91
doppelte Buchführung (E. Bleuler) (D) ... 91
doppelte Orientierung (D) ... 80
doppelte Persönlichkeit (D) ... 80
double bind (G. Bateson) (E) ... 80
double bind theory (G. Bateson) (E) ... 69
double orientation (E) ... 79
double personality (E) ... 80
down regulation (E) ... 68
Down syndrome (E) ... 68
Drang (D) ... 55
draw-a-person test (E) ... 55
dream anxiety disorder (E) ... 102

dreamy state (H. Jackson) (E)	98
Drehschwindel (D)	11
dressing apraxia (E)	71
drinking bout (E)	105
drive (E)	103
dromomania (E)	83
drowsiness (E)	26
Druckvision (D)	1
drug abuse (E)	101
drug addiction (E)	101
drug dependence (ICD-9) (E)	101
drug-induced extrapyramidal symptoms (E)	101
drug-induced mental disorder (E)	101
drug interaction (E)	101
drug intoxication (E)	101
drug therapy (E)	101
drug withdrawal syndrome (E)	101
drunkenness (E)	99
dual-role transvestism (E)	104
due to general medical condition (E)	20
duration of untreated psychosis (DUP) (E)	61
Durcharbeitung (S. Freud) (D)	74
Durchgangssyndrom (H. H. Wieck) (D)	74
dying patient (E)	104
dynamic psychiatry (E)	103
dysarthria (E)	30
dysdiadochokinesis (E)	94
dysesthesia (E)	5
dysgraphia (E)	50
dyskinesia (E)	41
dyslexia (E)	78
dysmetria (E)	66
dysmnesia (E)	17
dysmorphophobia (E)	45

dysorexia（E）	50
dysosmophobia（E）	1
dyspareunia（E）	57
dysphagia（E）	9
dysphoria（E）	91
dysphoric mania（E）	91
dysprosody（E）	7, 42
dysrhythmic migrane（E）	104
dyssomnia（E）	55
dysthymia（E）	20
dysthymic disorder（E）	20
dystonia（E）	41
early infantile autism（L. Kanner）（E）	65
early morning awakening（E）	66
early psychosis（E）	65
eating disorder（E）	63
écho de la lecture（F）	78
écho de la pensée（F）	31
echolalia（E）	85
echomimia（E）	85
echopraxia（E）	85
echo symptom（E）	85
echte Halluzination（D）	54
echter Wahn（D）	54
Echteschizophrenie（D）	54
ecmnesia（E）	52
ecmnésie（F）	52
ecstasy（E）	31
educational treatment（E）	73
EEG topography（E）	82
effeminatio（L）	50
ego（E）	37
ego boundary（E）	37
ego-dystonic（E）	37

egogram（E） ……………………………………………………………… 8
ego ideal（E） …………………………………………………………… 38
ego identity（E. H. Erikson）（E） ………………………………… 38
egorrh(o)ea symptoms（藤縄昭）（E） …………………………… 38
ego-syntonic（E） ……………………………………………………… 38
Eidetiker（E. R. Jaensch）（D） …………………………………… 73
eidetische Anlage（E. R. Jaensch）（D） ………………………… 73
Eifersuchtswahn（D） ………………………………………………… 42
Eigenbeziehung（D） ………………………………………………… 40
Einfühlen（D） ………………………………………………………… 15
einfühlendes Verstehen（D） ……………………………………… 15
Einfühlung（D） ……………………………………………………… 15
Einheitspsychose（W. Griesinger, H. W. Neuman）（D） ……… 70
Einschlaferlebnis（D） ……………………………………………… 81
Einschlafmittel（D） ………………………………………………… 56
Einsicht（D） …………………………………………………………… 77
Einstellungsstörung（D） …………………………………………… 33
elder abuse（E） …………………………………………………… 106
elderly health care facility（E） ………………………………… 106
elective mutism（E） ………………………………………………… 64
Electra complex（E） ………………………………………………… 9
electroconvulsive therapy（ECT）（E） …………………………… 75
electroconvulsive treatment（E） ………………………………… 75
electroencephalogram（E） ………………………………………… 82
electroencephalography（EEG）（E） …………………………… 82
elektiver Mutismus（M. Tramer）（D） …………………………… 64
Elektroschocktherapie（ES）（D） ………………………………… 75
elementary hallucination（E） …………………………………… 102
elementary seizure（E） …………………………………………… 102
Embryonalstellung（D） …………………………………………… 67
emergency hospitalization（E） …………………………………… 9
emergency psychiatry（E） …………………………………… 20, 58
emotion（E） …………………………………………………………… 48
Emotion（D） …………………………………………………………… 48

émotion （F） …… 48
emotionale Depression （K. Schneider）（D） …… 49
emotional incontinence （E） …… 49
emotionally unstable personality disorder （E） …… 49
Emotionslähmung （D） …… 49
Emotionsstupor （D） …… 48
empathy （E） …… 15
empirische Erbprognose （D） …… 26
empty nest syndrome （E） …… 14
encephalitis （E） …… 82
encephalitis japonica （L） …… 80
encephalography （E） …… 82
encopresis （E） …… 6
endocrinological psychiatry （E） …… 79
endogenous （E） …… 78
endogenous depression （E） …… 79
endogenous psychosis （E） …… 79
endokrines Psychosyndrom （M. Bleuler）（D） …… 79
endoreaktive Dysthymie （H. J. Weitbrecht）（D） …… 79
énergie psychique （F） …… 55
engram （E） …… 17
Engramm （R. Semon）（D） …… 17
Entartung （D） …… 94
Enterozoenwahn （D） …… 73
Entfremdung （D） …… 66
Entfremdungsgefühl （D） …… 40, 66
Enthemmung （D） …… 103
Entlastungsdepression （W. Schulte）（D） …… 79
Entmündigung （D） …… 87
Entwurzelungsdepression （H. Bürger-Prinz）（D） …… 81
Entziehung （D） …… 104
Entziehungskur （D） …… 24
enuresis （E） …… 6
enuresis diurnal （L） …… 72

enuresis nocturna (L)	100
Epilepsie (D)	75
épilepsie (F)	75
epilepsy (E)	75
epileptic psychosis (E)	75
epileptic twilight state (E)	75
epileptischer Dämmerzustand (D)	75
epileptoid (E)	75
Epileptoid (D)	75
epileptoid personality (E)	105
epileptology (E)	75
episode (E)	66
episodic memory (E. Tulving) (E)	9
episodischer Dämmerzustand (D)	65
equivalent (E)	76
Erbanlage (D)	6
Erbprognose (D)	6
erectile disorder (ED) (E)	95
ereuthophobia (E)	62
Erfindungswahn (D)	85
ergothérapie (F)	36
Erinnerungsfälschung (D)	74
Erinnerungshalluzination (D)	73
Erinnerungsillusion (D)	73
Erinnerungstäuschung (D)	74
Erklärungswahn (C. Wernicke) (D)	63
Erlebnisreaktion (D)	67
Erlebnisverarbeitung (D)	67
Erleuchtungserlebnis (D)	37
erogenous zone (E)	57
erotomania (E)	38, 105
érotomanie (F)	38
érotomanie (G. G. de Clérambault) (F)	105
Ersatzbildung (D)	68

Erschöpfungsdepression (P. Kielholz) (D) ……………………………………… 49
Erschöpfungsneurose (D) ……………………………………………………… 49
Erschwerung der Wortfindung (D) …………………………………………… 15
Erwartungsangst (D) …………………………………………………………… 102
Erwartungsneurose (D) ………………………………………………………… 102
erythrophobia (E) ……………………………………………………………… 62
Es (D) …………………………………………………………………………… 9
escape (E) ……………………………………………………………………… 77
essential tremor (E) …………………………………………………………… 96
état crépusculaire (F) ………………………………………………………… 100
état oniroïde (F) ……………………………………………………………… 98
ethnopsychiatry (E) …………………………………………………………… 97
eugenics (E) …………………………………………………………………… 102
euphoria (E) …………………………………………………………………… 69
euthanasia (E) ………………………………………………………………… 4
event-related potential (E) …………………………………………………… 41
evidence-based medicine (EBM) (E) ………………………………………… 9
evolution (H. Jackson) (E) …………………………………………………… 51
examining oneself (E) ………………………………………………………… 97
excessive sleepness (E) ……………………………………………………… 81
executive function (E) ………………………………………………………… 55
exhibitionism (E) ……………………………………………………………… 106
existentielle Depression (H. Häfner) (D) …………………………………… 42
Existenzanalyse (D) …………………………………………………………… 42
exogene Prädilektionstypen (K. Bonhoeffer) (D) …………………………… 10
exogene Reaktionstypen (K. Bonhoeffer) (D) ……………………………… 10
exogenous predilection type (E) ……………………………………………… 10
exogenous psychosis (E) ……………………………………………………… 10
exogenous reaction type (E) ………………………………………………… 10
expansiver Wahn (D) …………………………………………………………… 34
expectation anxiety (E) ……………………………………………………… 102
experimental neurosis (E) …………………………………………………… 42
experimental psychosis (E) …………………………………………………… 42
expertise psychiatrique (F) …………………………………………………… 58

explanatory delusion (E) 63
explicit memory (E) 10, 28
Explosible (Psychopathen) (K. Schneider) (D) 84
expressed emotion (EE) (E) 16
expressive aphasia (E) 89
expressive language disorder (ICD-10, DSM-III-R) (E) 89
extensibilité (F) 55
extracampine hallucination (E) 4
extraversion (E) 10
eyedness (E) 17
Fabulieren (D) 36
facial apraxia (E) 16
facial tic (E) 16
facility for training in daily life of the person with mental disorder (E) 59
factitious disorder (DSM-III) (E) 23
facultive symptom (E) 81
Fahr disease (E) 90
failure of genital response (E) 62
false memory (syndrome) (E) 23
family denial delusion (E) 13
family dynamics (E) 13
family psychiatry (E) 13
family schism (E) 13
family therapy (E) 13
family violence (E) 13
family with high expressed emotion (EE) (E) 30
Fanatiker (D) 22
Fanatische (Psychopathen) (K. Schneider) (D) 13, 22
Farbenagnosie (D) 38
Farbenhören (D) 38
fasciculation (E) 63
fastidium (E) 94
Faxensyndrom (D) 76
fear of emitting body odor (E) 40

F

fear of eye-to-eye confrontation (E) ······ 40
febrile convulsion (E) ······ 81
feeding disorder (E) ······ 94
feeling (E) ······ 15
feeling of inferiority (E) ······ 105
feeling of insufficiency (E) ······ 92
feeling of omnipotence (E) ······ 65
Fehlleistung (D) ······ 36
female orgasmic disorder (E) ······ 50
feminization (E) ······ 50
festinating gait (E) ······ 13
festination (E) ······ 13
fetal alcohol syndrome (E) ······ 67
fetal period (E) ······ 68
fetishism (E) ······ 90
fever therapy (E) ······ 85
fibrillation (E) ······ 63
Fieberdelirium (D) ······ 81
Fiebertherapie (D) ······ 85
field of consciousness (E) ······ 5
filial therapy (E) ······ 90
finger agnosia (E) ······ 46, 102
finger sucking (E) ······ 102
first rank symptoms (E) ······ 5
fixation (E) ······ 34
fixed idea (E) ······ 34
Fixierung (D) ······ 34
flaccid paralysis (E) ······ 38
flapping tremor (E) ······ 84
flashback phenomenon (E) ······ 93
flexibilitas cerea (L) ······ 106
flight into illness (E) ······ 43
flight of ideas (E) ······ 16
flooding (E) ······ 93

Flucht（D）	77
Flucht in die Krankheit（D）	43
fluent aphasia（E）	104
focal motor seizure（E）	48
focal seizure（E）	48
focal symptom（E）	48, 66
focusing（E）	91
folie à deux（F）	92
folie alterne（F）	32
folie circulaire（J-P. Falret）（F）	47
folie de doute（F）	24
folie discordante（P. Chaslin）（F）	92
folie raisonnante（F）	104
fonction du réel（P. Janet）（F）	28
food refusal（E）	24
forced crying（E）	23
forced grasping（E）	22
forced laughing（E）	23
forced laughter（E）	23
forced weeping（E）	23
forensic psychiatry（E）	44
formed hallucination（E）	102
foster employer system（臺弘）（E）	50
foster home care（E）	36
fox possession（E）	19
Fragesucht（D）	43
fraktionierte Aktivhypnose（E. Kretschmer）（D）	93
free association（E）	46
free-floating anxiety（E）	92
free walking（E）	88
Frégoli syndrome（E）	93
Fremdheitserlebnis（D）	98
Fremdneurose（J. H. Schultz）（D）	5
frigidity（E）	105

frontal lobe syndrome (E) ······ 65
frontal lobotomy (W. Freeman & J. W. Watts) (E) ······ 65
frontotemporal dementia (FTD) (E) ······ 64
frontotemporal dementia and parkinsonism linked to chromosome 17 (E) ······ 9
frontotemporal lobar degeneration (FTLD) (E) ······ 64
frozen gait (E) ······ 56
frustration (E) ······ 103
fugue (E, F) ······ 79
functional hallucination (E) ······ 19
functional psychosis (E) ······ 19
Fundamental Law for Countermeasures Concerning Mentally and Physically Handicapped Persons (E) ······ 53
Funktionswandel (V. v. Weizsäcker) (D) ······ 19
gain from illness (E) ······ 43
gait disturbance (E) ······ 95
Galgenhumor (D) ······ 56
Ganserscher Dämmerzustand (D) ······ 15
Ganser syndrome (E) ······ 15
Ganzheitsstörung (D) ······ 64
Gaucher disease (E) ······ 33
Gedächtnis (D) ······ 17
Gedächtnishalluzination (D) ······ 17
Gedächtnisstörung (D) ······ 17
Gedankenarmut (D) ······ 31
Gedankenausbreitung (D) ······ 31
Gedankenbeeinflußung (D) ······ 39
Gedankendrängen (D) ······ 39
Gedankenecho (D) ······ 31
Gedankeneningebung (D) ······ 31
Gedankenentzug (D) ······ 31
Gedankengang (D) ······ 51
Gedankengangstörung (D) ······ 51
Gedankenlautwerden (G. Störring) (D) ······ 31
Gedankensichtbarwerden (K. Halbey) (D) ······ 31

Gedankensprung (D)	39
Gedankenverstandenwerden (D)	31
Gefühl (D)	15
Gefühlsabstumpfung (D)	16
Gegenhalten (D)	74, 85
Gegenstandsbewußtsein (D)	67
Gegenübertragung (D)	20
Gegenzwang (D)	67
Gehirnkarte (D)	82
Gehirnpathologie (D)	82
Gehörshalluzination (D)	29
Geistesstörung (D)	59
geistiges Ich (D)	58
Gelegenheitsanfälle (D)	48
Geltungsbedürfnis (D)	29
Geltungsbedürftige (Psychopathen) (K. Schneider) (D)	28
gemachtes Erlebnis (D)	36
gemachtes Phänomen (D)	36
Gemütlose (Psychopathen) (K. Schneider) (D)	48
gender identity (E)	62
gender identity disorder (E)	62
general adaptation syndrome (H. Selye) (E)	86
general hospital psychiatry (E)	65
generalized anxiety disorder (E)	65
generalized convalsion (E)	68
generalized convulsive seizure (E)	65
generalized epilepsy (E)	65
general paralysis (E)	53
general paresis (E)	53
Generationspsychose (D)	57
genetisches Verstehen (D)	84
genital stage (E)	57
genotype (E)	5
genuine epilepsy (E)	54

gereizte Manie (D)	6
geriatric psychiatry (E)	105
gerichtliche Psychiatrie (D)	44
gerontophilia (E)	106
Gerstmann syndrome (E)	27
Geruchshalluzination (D)	27
Geschäftsfähigkeit (D)	30
Geschlechtskälte (D)	105
Geschmackshalluzination (D)	29
Geschmacksillusion (D)	36
Gesichtshalluzination (D)	28
Gesichtsschneiden (D)	88
Gestaltfunktion (D)	26
Gestaltwandel (D)	26
gestural automatism (E)	97
Gilles de la Tourette syndrome (E)	78
global aphasia (E)	64
globus hystericus (L)	88
glossolalia (E)	41
glue sniffing (E)	101
gnash (E)	83
going my way behavior (E)	106
graft schizophrenia (E)	63
grand hystérie (J. M. Charcot) (F)	68
grandiose delusion (E)	34
grand mal (F)	68
graphology (E)	88
grasp reflex (E)	82
Greifreflex (D)	83
grief therapy (E)	25
grimace (E)	38
grimas (E)	38
Grimasse (D)	38
Grimassieren (D)	38

Größenwahn (D)	34
group psychotherapy (E)	46
Grübelsucht (D)	64
Grundstimung (D)	19
Grundstörung (D)	20
guardian (E)	30
guidance of daily activity (E)	56
guilt feeling (E)	35
Gulf-War syndrome (E)	106
gustatory hallucination (E)	29
gustatory seizure (E)	97
gyn(a)ephobia (E)	50
habilitation (E)	85
habitual criminal (E)	48
Haftpsychose (D)	30
Haftreaktion (D)	30
Haftstupor (D)	30
Halbschlafdenken (D)	86
halfway house (E)	85
hallucination (E) (F)	27
hallucination négative (F)	6
hallucination of equilibrium (E)	93
hallucination psychique (J. Baillarger) (F)	58
hallucination psychomotrice verbale (J. Séglas) (F)	28
hallucinatory seizure (E)	27
hallucinogen (E)	27
hallucinogen abuse (E)	27
hallucinogen dependence (E)	27
hallucinogen-induced anxiety disorders (E)	27
hallucinogen-induced disorders (E)	27
hallucinogen-induced mood disorders (E)	27
hallucinogen-induced psychotic disorders (E)	27
hallucinogen intoxication (E)	27
hallucinogen intoxication delirium (E)	27

hallucinogen persisting perception disorder（flashbacks）（E） 27
hallucinogen-related disorders（DSM-IV）（E） 27
hallucinogen use disorders（E） 27
hallucinose pédonculaire（J. Lhermitte）（F） 72
Halluzination（D） 27
Halluzinose（C. Wernicke）（D） 27
Haltlose（E. Kraepelin）（D） 26
Haltungsstereotypie（D） 48
Hamilton Rating Scale for Depression（E） 85
handedness（E） 17
handicap（E） 44
Handlungsfähigkeit（D） 30
hang-over effect（E） 100
haptic hallucination（E） 29
Hasegawa Dementia Scale（HDS，改訂版 HDS-R）（E） 84
Hauptklage（D） 46
head retraction reflex（E） 76
Health and Medical Service Law for the Aged（E） 106
héautoscopie（F） 40
Heautoskopie（D） 40
heavy work stage（Morita therapy）（E） 45
hebephrenia（E） 83
hebephrenic schizophrenia（E） 83
Hebephrenie（E. Hecker）（D） 83
Heboidophrenie（L. Kahlbaum）（D） 105
Heilpädagogik（D） 73
Heimwehrreaktion（D） 22
Heller syndrome（E） 94
hemianopsia（E） 86
hemiasomatognosia（E） 86
hemiballism（E） 94
hemicrania（E） 94
hemiplegia（E） 94
Hemmung（D） 30, 57

hepatic encephalopathy （E） ……………………………………………………… 16
hepatocerebral disease （E） ……………………………………………………… 16
hepatocerebral disease of Inose type （E） ……………………………………… 6
hepatolenticular degeneration （Wilson disease） （E） ……………………… 16
Herdsymptom （D） ………………………………………………………………… 66
herpes simplex encephalitis （E） ………………………………………………… 70
Herzneurose （D） …………………………………………………………………… 54
heterosexuality （E） ………………………………………………………………… 5
high risk study （E） ………………………………………………………………… 30
Hintergrundreaktion （D） ………………………………………………………… 83
Hirnarteriosklerose （D） …………………………………………………………… 82
hirnlokales Psychosyndrom （M. Bleuler） （D） ……………………………… 82
Hirnlues （D） ………………………………………………………………………… 82
histrionic personality disorder （DSM-III） （E） ……………………………… 9
Hochstapler （D） …………………………………………………………………… 53
höheres Gefühl （D） ……………………………………………………………… 48
holding （E） ………………………………………………………………………… 96
holism （E） ………………………………………………………………………… 64
holothymer Wahn （D） …………………………………………………………… 64
home care （E） ……………………………………………………………………… 35
home violence （E） ………………………………………………………………… 14
homilophobia （E） ………………………………………………………………… 31
homonymous hemianopsia （E） ………………………………………………… 78
homosexuality （E） ………………………………………………………………… 77
Hörstummheit （D） ………………………………………………………………… 72
hospice （E） ………………………………………………………………………… 95
hospitalism （E） ……………………………………………………………… 41, 95
hospital psychiatry （E） …………………………………………………………… 89
Humoralpathologie （D） …………………………………………………………… 67
humoral pathology （E） …………………………………………………………… 67
hump （E） ………………………………………………………………………… 104
Huntington disease （E） …………………………………………………………… 85
hydrocephalus （E） ………………………………………………………………… 55
hyperarousal （E） …………………………………………………………………… 12

hyperästhetisch-emotionaler Schwächezustand (K. Bonhoeffer) (D) 14
hyperbulia (E) 6
Hyperbulie (D) 6
hypercinesia(-sis) (E) 8
hyperesthesia (E) 14
hypergraphia (S. G. Waxman & N. Geschwind) (E) 13
hyperkinesia(-sis) (E) 8
hyperkinesis (E) 69
hyperkinetic disorder (ICD-10) (E) 69
hypermetamorphosis (E) 94
hypermnesia (E) 17
Hypermnesie (D) 17
hyperorexia (E) 50
hyperpathia (E) 89
Hyperpathie (D) 89
hypersexuality (E) 62
hypersomnia (E) 14, 56
hyperthymia (E) 19
Hyperthymische (Psychopathen) (K. Schneider) (D) 85
hyperventilation syndrome (E) 12
hypesthesia (E) 15
hypnagogic hallucination (E) 80
hypnoanalysis (E) 36
hypnopompic hallucination (E) 46
hypnosis (E) 35
hypnotherapy (E) 36
hypnotics (E) 56
hypoactive sexual desire disorder (E) 62
hypobulia (E) 6
Hypobulie (D) 6
hypobulischer Mechanismus (E. Kretschmer) (D) 13
hypochondriacal delusion (E) 52
hypochondriacal temperament (森田正馬) (E) 89
hypochondriasis (E) 52

Hypochondrie (D)	52
hypochondrischer Wahn (D)	52
hypocinesia(-sis) (E)	8
hypofrontality (E)	65
hypokinesia(-sis) (E)	8
hypomania (E)	26
hypomanic episode (E)	26
hypomnesia (E)	17
Hypomnesie (D)	17
hyponoischer Mechanismus (E. Kretschmer) (D)	13
hypoprosexia (E)	72
hyposexuality (E)	62
hypothymia (E)	20
hypotonia (E)	24
hypsarythmia (E)	89
hysteresis (E)	104
hysteria (E)	88
hysterical character (E)	88
hysterical personality disorder (ICD-9) (E)	88
hysterical psychosis (E)	88
hysterischer Bogen (D)	88
hystéro-épilepsie (F)	88
hysteroepilepsy (E)	88
iatrogenic disease (E)	4
iatrogenic neurosis (E)	4
Ich (D)	37
Ich-Anachorese (W. Th. Winkler) (D)	38
Ichbewußtsein (D)	37
Icherlebnis (D)	38
Ichgefühl (D)	37
Ichgrenzen (P. Federn) (D)	37
Ichhaftigkeit (D)	38
Ichstörung (D)	38
ictal (E)	95

ictal automatism（E）	95
ictal stupor（E）	75, 95
id（E）	9
idealization（E）	104
idea of suicide（E）	40
ideational apraxia（E）	16
idée délirante（F）	99
Ideenarmut（D）	16
Ideenassoziation（D）	16
Ideenflucht（D）	16
identification（E）	75
identity crisis（E. H. Erikson）（E）	75
identity diffusion syndrome（E. H. Erikson）（E）	75
ideomotor apraxia（E）	16
illness（E）	43
illusion（E）	36
illusion de Frégoli（P. Courbon & G. Fail）（F）	12
illusion des sosies（J. Capgras & J. Reboul-Lachaux）（F）	8
Imago（C. G. Jung）（D）	6
immediate memory（E）	66
Immodithymie（Immobilithymie）（下田光造）（D）	46
implicit memory（E）	79
impotence（E）	62
impressibility（E）	20
impulse（E）	85
impulse-control disorder（E）	49
impulsion（E）	55
impulsive act（E）	48
impulsive Handlung（D）	48
Impulsiv-petit-mal（D. Janz）（D）	48
imu（E）	6
Imudo（D）	6
inadequate personality（E）	92
Inanitionspsychose（D）	17

inattention (E)	92
incest (E)	24
incidence (E)	84
incoherence (E)	51
incoherence of thought (E)	40
individual psychotherapy (E)	33
induced delusional disorder (ICD-10) (E)	16
induced psychosis (E)	16
induzierte Psychose (D)	16
infant home (E)	80
infantile convulsion (E)	81
infantile psychiatry (E)	81
infantile spasms (F. A. & E. L. Gibbs) (E)	75
infantilism (E)	49
Infektionspsychose (D)	16
informed consent (E)	7
inhalant (E)	21
inhalant abuse (E)	21
inhalant dependency (E)	21
inhalant-induced disorder (E)	21
inhalant-related disorder (E)	21
inhalant use disorder (E)	21
inhibition (E)	57
inhibition of thought (E)	39
initial cry (E)	50
Initialschrei (D)	50
initiation ceremony (E)	74
Initiativelosigkeit (D)	44
Inkohärenz (D)	39, 51
inner speech (E)	79
inpatient (E)	80
inpatients with social reasons (E)	44
Inselaphasie (D)	77
insight (E)	77

insight into disease (E) 89
insight therapy (E) 77
insomnia (E) 92
instinct (E) 96
instinct of self-preservation (E) 38
institutionalism (E) 41
institutionalization (E) 41
institutional neurosis (E) 41
institutional rehabilitation (E) 41
insulin-coma treatment (E) 6
Insulinkomabehandlung (M. Sakel) (D) 6
Insulinschocktherapie (D) 6
integrated education (E) 76
intellectualization (E) 71
intelligence (E) 71
intelligence quotient (IQ) (E) 71
intelligence test (E) 71
Intelligenz (D) 71
Intelligenzalter (D) 71
Intelligenzprüfung (D) 71
intensive care unit psychosis, ICU psychosis (E) 46
intensive care unit syndrome (E) 1
intention tremor (E) 19
interdiction (E) 87
inter-ictal dysphoric syndrome (E) 95
inter-ictal psychosis (E) 95
intermittent awakening (E) 72
intermittent explosive disorder (DSM-IV) (E) 15
International Classification of Diseases (ICD) (WHO) (E) 33
internuclear ophthalmoplegia (E) 12
interpretation (E) 10
interprétation (F) 10
intoxication psychosis (E) 72
Intoxikationspsychose (D) 72

intractable depression (E) 79
intramural remission (E) 7
intrapsychische Ataxie (E. Stransky) (D) 55
introjection (E) 79
Introjektion (D) 79
introspection (E) 79
introversion (E) 79
Invokationspsychose (森田正馬) (D) 19
involuntary hospitalization ordered by prefectural governor (E) 66
involuntary movement (E) 91
involutional melancholia (E) 67
involutional psychosis (E) 67
Involutionsmelancholie (D) 67
irresponsibility (E) 54
irritability (E) 5, 39
irritable weakness (E) 39
island aphasia (E) 77
Iteration (D) 86
Jacksonian march (E) 45
Jacksonian seizure (E) 45
Jacksonism (E) 45
jamais vu (F) 97
Japan Association of Community Workshop for Disabled Persons (E) 22
Japanese Association of Neuro-Psychiatric Clinics (E) 80
Japanese Association of Psychiatric Hospitals (E) 80
japanese encephalitis (E) 80
Japanese Society of Psychiatry and Neurology (JSPN) (E) 80
Japan Federation for Mental Health and Welfare (E) 80
jargon aphasia (E) 45
jaw jerk (E) 12
jet lag syndrome (E) 40
joint interview (E) 77
juvenile absence epilepsy (E) 45
juvenile Alzheimer disease (E) 45

juvenile myoclonic epilepsy (E) 45
juvenile paresis (E) 45
Kampfparanoia (D) 77
Kastrationsangst (D) 24
Katastrophenreaktion (K. Goldstein) (D) 83
katathymer Wahn (D) 16
Katatonie (D) 24
kategoriales Verhalten (K. Goldstein) (D) 86
Kaufsucht (D) 103
kausaler Zusammenhang (K. Jaspers) (D) 6
kausales Erklären (D) 6
keraunophobia (E) 6
Kernneurose (J. H. Schultz) (D) 72
Kinderneurose (D) 43
Kinderpsychiatrie (D) 43
Kinderschizophrenie (D) 43
kindling (E) 24
kinésie paradoxale (F) 98
kinesthetic hallucination (E) 8
kinetic family drawing (KFD) (E) 77
Kipprezidiv (D) 102
Klangassoziation (D) 10
Kleidungsapraxie (D) 71
Kleine-Levin syndrome (E) 25
kleine Psychotherapie (D) 48
Kleinheitswahn (D) 88
Klinefelter syndrome (E) 25
klonischer Krampf (D) 16
Klüver-Bucy syndrome (E) 25
Knick der Persönlichkeitsentwicklung (D) 52
Kohs blocks test (E) 34
Kollathymie (W. Enke) (D) 81
kollektives Unbewußtes (C. G. Jung) (D) 92
Koma (D) 35

Kommotionspsychose（D） ……………………………………………………… 82
Komplex（D） …………………………………………………………………… 35
komplizierter Rausch（D） …………………………………………………… 91
komplizierte Schmollen（D） ………………………………………………… 91
Konfabulation（D） ……………………………………………………………… 36
konstruktive Apraxie（D） …………………………………………………… 31
Kontrollzwang（D） ……………………………………………………………… 12
Konzentrationslagersyndrome（D） ………………………………………… 22
koro（E） ………………………………………………………………………… 34
Körper-Ich（D） ………………………………………………………………… 54
körperlich begründbare Psychose（K. Schneider）（D） ………………… 55
Körperschema（D） ……………………………………………………………… 54
Korsakoff psychosis（E） ……………………………………………………… 34
Korsakoff syndrome（E） ……………………………………………………… 34
Kotschmieren（D） ……………………………………………………………… 78
Kraepelin disease（E） ………………………………………………………… 25
Kraepelinische Krankheit（D） ……………………………………………… 25
Krampf（D） ……………………………………………………………………… 26
Krampfanfall（D） ……………………………………………………………… 26
Krampfbehandlung（D） ……………………………………………………… 26
Krankenhauspsychiatrie（D） ………………………………………………… 89
Krankheitseinheit（D） ………………………………………………………… 42
Krankheitseinsicht（D） ……………………………………………………… 89
Krankheitsgefühl（D） ………………………………………………………… 89
Krankheitsgewinn（D） ………………………………………………………… 43
Kriegsneurose（D） ……………………………………………………………… 64
Kurihama Alcoholism Screening Test（KAST）（E） …………………… 25
Kurzschlußreaktion（D） ……………………………………………………… 70
labor resettlement system（E） ……………………………………………… 50
Lachschlag（D） ………………………………………………………………… 106
lack of criminal responsibility（E） ………………………………………… 62
lacunar dementia（E） ………………………………………………………… 96
Laktationspsychose（D） ……………………………………………………… 47
Landau-Kleffner syndrome（E） …………………………………………… 103

landscape montage technique (E)	90
läppisch (D)	38
larvierte (maskierte) Depression (D)	14
latah (E)	103
late catatonia (E)	71
late depression (E)	71
latency period (E)	64
latent schizophrenia (E)	64, 65
latent schizophreniform reaction (E)	64
Latenzperiode (D)	64
late paraphrenia (M. Roth) (E)	71
late schizophrenia (E)	71
Laurence-Moon-Biedl syndrome (E)	106
Law for Supporting Persons with Developmental Disabilities (E)	84
law for the welfare of the physically handicapped (E)	54
laziness of thinking (E)	39
lead-pipe rigidity (E)	9
learning difficulty (LD) (E)	12
learning disability (LD) (E)	12
leeres Lachen (D)	25
leibhaftige Bewußtheit (D)	42
Leibhaftigkeit (D)	42
Leidensdruck (D)	42
Lennox-Gastaut syndrome (E)	105
lepraphobia (E)	103
leptosomatic (E)	101
le réel (J. Lacan) (F)	28
lesbian (E)	105
Lesch-Nyhan syndrome (E)	105
lethal catatonia (E)	71
lethargy (E)	44
liaison psychiatry (E)	103
libido (E)	104
Lichtphonismus (D)	30

Lidschlußapraxie (D) 93
Liebeswahn (D) 105
Liepmann phenomenon (E) 104
life cycle (E) 103
life event (E) 103
life history (E) 57
life stage (E) 103
light reflex (E) 67
light work stage (Morita therapy) (E) 26
lilliputian hallucination (E) 34
l'imaginaire (J. Lacan) (F) 66
limbic system (E) 68
limb-kinetic apraxia (E) 41
Lippensprache (D) 53
literal paraphasia (E) 41
living learning (臺弘) (E) 57
living will (E) 104
lobotomy (E) 106
local council on mental health and welfare (E) 71
local symptom (E) 24
locked-in syndrome (E) 78
logoclonia (E) 28
Logoklonie (D) 28
logorrh(o)ea (E) 34
Logotherapie (V. E. Frankl) (D) 106
Lokalisationslehre (D) 68
longitudinal study (E) 46
Long-term care insurance (E) 10
long term memory (E) 73
loosening of association (E) 105
loss of consciousness (E) 5
loss of initiative (E) 44
Lügen (D) 24
lupus psychosis (E) 105

L～M

Lustmord（D）	11
Lustprinzip（S. Freud）（D）	11
Lust-Unlust-Prinzip（D）	11
lycanthropy（E）	9
lying（E）	24
lypémanie（E. Esquirol）（F）	104
macrocephaly（E）	68
macrographia（E）	67
macropsia（E）	67
magical thinking（E）	46
magnetic resonance angiography（E）	9
magnetic resonance angiography（MRA）（E）	38
magnetic resonance imaging（E）	9
magnetic resonance imaging（MRI）（E）	38
magnetic resonance spectroscopy（MRS）（E）	38
magnétisme animal（F）	77
magnetoencephalography（MEG）（E）	82
major depression（DSM-III）（E）	66
major depressive disorder（DSM-IV）（E）	67
maladie créatrice（H. F. Ellenberger）（F）	66
maladjustment（E）	92
maladjustment reaction（ICD-9）（E）	92
Malariakur（D）	96
malingering（E）	37
mandala（E）	97
mania（E）	66
manic defense（E）	66
manic-depressive psychosis（E）	65
manic episode（DSM-IV-TR）（E）	66
manic switch（E）	66
Manie（D）	66
manie（F）	66
Manieriertheit（D）	106
manisch-depressive Irresein（D）	65

mannerism（E）	106
map of cerebral cortex（E）	82
Marchiafava-Bignami disease（E）	96
marital schism（T. Lidz）（E）	90
marital skew（T. Lidz）（E）	90
masculinization（E）	70
masked depression（E）	14
masked epilepsy（E）	14
masked face（E）	14
Maskengesicht（D）	14
mask-like face（E）	14
masochism（E）	87
Massenhysterie（D）	46
mass hysteria（E）	46
masturbation（E）	96
maternal deprivation（E）	95
maternity blues（E）	96
mathematics disorder（DSM-IV）（E）	37
measures taken for the preservation of public security（E）	94
Medea complex（E）	99
medical psychiatry（E）	54
megacephaly（E）	68
megalencephaly（E）	24
megalomania（E）	34
mégalomanie（F）	34
mehrdimensionale Diagnostik（E. Kretschmer）（D）	69
Meige syndrome（E）	98
Meinhaftigkeit（D）	40
melancholia（E）	99
melancholia attonita（L）	38
melancholic features（DSM-IV）（E）	99
Melancholie（D）	99
mélancholie（F）	99
mémoire（F）	17

M

mémoire sociale（J. Delay）（F）	44
memory（E）	17
memory trace（E）	17
mensonge（F）	24
mental age（MA）（E）	60
mental clinic（E）	58
mental deficiency（E）	60
mental deterioration（E）	60
mental disorder（E）	59
mental health（E）	61
Mental Health and Welfare Act（E）	61
mental health and welfare center（E）	61
mental health center（E）	61
Mental Health Law（E）	61
mental hospital（E）	58
Mental Hospital Act（E）	61
mental hygiene（E）	58
mentally handicapped person who engages illegal conduct and comes under the protection of the law（E）	50
mental preoccupation（Morita therapy）（E）	79
mental retardation（E）	60, 71
Merkfähigkeit（D）	20
Merkprüfung（三宅鑛一）（D）	97
Merkschwäche（D）	20
metachromatic leukodystrophy（MLD）（E）	5
metamorphopsia（E）	94
metamorphotischer Wahn（D）	94
metapsychology（E）	99
microcephaly（ia）（E）	49
micr[o]encephaly[-lia]（E）	106
micrographia（E）	48
microgyria（E）	49
micropsia（E）	48
migrane（E）	94

mild cognitive impairment (MCI) (E) 26
mild depression (E) 26
mild mental retardation (E) 60
Milieureaktion (D) 15
milieu therapy (E) 15
Minamata disease (E) 97
Minderwertigkeitsgefühl (D) 105
mind reading (E) 31
minimal brain dysfunction (MBD) (E) 87
Minnesota Multiphasic Personality Inventory (MMPI) (E) 97
minor anomaly (E) 96
mirror foci (E) 22
Mischpsychose (D) 34
Mischzustand (W. Weygandt) (D) 34
misidentification (E) 55
mismatch negativity (E) 97
Mißbrauch (D) 103
Mitfühlen (D) 22
mitochondrial encephalomyopathy (E) 97
mixed affective disorder (E) 15
mixed anxiety and depressive disorder (E) 35
mixed disorder of conduct and emotion (ICD-10) (E) 66
mixed psychosis (E) 34
mixed receptive-expressive language disorder (DSM-IV) (E) 47
mixed specific developmental disorder (E) 34
mixed state (E) 34
mixed transcortical aphasia (E) 34
Miyake recent memory scale (E) 97
mnemic function (E) 17
modeling (E) 100
moderate mental retardation (E) 60, 72
modified electroconvulsive therapy (m-ECT) (E) 46
moi (F) 37
monolog (ue) (E) 78

monomania (E) 100
monomanie (E. Esquirol) (F) 100
monopolare Depression (D) 70
mood (affective) disorder (E) 20
mood congruent psychotic features (E) 20
mood disorder with rapid cycling (DSM-IV) (E) 89
mood episode (E) 19
mood incongruent psychotic features (E) 20
mood stabilizer (E) 19
moral therapy (E) 100
moral treatment (E) 100
morbidity risk (E) 104
moria (E) 10, 100
Morita therapy (E) 100
morphinism (E) 100
mothering (E) 95
Motilitätspsychose (C. Wernicke) (D) 8
motivation (E) 76
motor aphasia (E) 8
motor impersistence (E) 8
motor neglect (E) 8
motor skills disorder (DSM-IV) (E) 8
mourning work (E) 87
multiaxial evaluation (E) 69
multidimensional diagnosis (E) 69
multi-infarct dementia (E) 69
multiple personality (E) 69
multiple personality disorder (ICD-10, DSM-III-R) (E) 69
multiple sclerosis (MS) (E) 69
multiple sleep latency test (E) 9
multiple sleep latency test (MSLT) (E) 56, 80
multiple spike complex (E) 68
multiple system atrophy (MSA) (E) 69
Munchausen syndrome (E) 97

Munchausen syndrome by proxy (E) 68
Münchhausen Syndrom (D) 97
muscle contraction headache (E) 24
musical hallucination (E) 10
musicogenic epilepsy (E) 10
musicolepsy (E) 10
music therapy (E) 10
Muskelsinnhalluzination (H. Cramer) (D) 24
mutism (E) 16
mutisme electif (F) 64
Mutismus (D) 16
myoclonic seizure (E) 97
myoclonus (E) 97
myoclonus epilepsy (E) 97
mysophobia (E) 91
mythomania (E) 24
mythomanie (E. Dupré) (F) 24
Nachahmungsautomatie (D) 100
Nachhallphänomen (D) 93
Nachtepilepsie (D) 101
Nackenstarre (D) 32
Nahrungsverweigerung (D) 24
Naikan therapy (E) 79
nail biting (E) 74
naming difficulty (E) 15
narcissism (E) 39
narcissistic personarity disorder (DSM-III) (E) 39
narcoanalysis (E) 96
narcolepsy (E) 79
narcotherapy (E) 96
narcotics anonymous (NA) (E) 96
narcotics intoxication (E) 96
narrative based medicine (E) 79
National Federation of Families with Mentaly Ill in Japan (E) 63

National Federation of Mental Health and Welfare Party in Japan："Minna Net"
 (E) ……………………………………………………………………………… 64
natürliche Selbstverständlichkeit（W. Blankenburg）(D) ……………………… 41
near(-)death experience (E) …………………………………………………… 104
Nebenwahn (D) ………………………………………………………………… 91
necrophilia (E) ………………………………………………………………… 41
necrotizing encephalitis (E) …………………………………………………… 8
negation (E) …………………………………………………………………… 89
negative hallucination (E) …………………………………………………… 6
negative symptoms (E) ……………………………………………………… 6
negativism (E) ………………………………………………………………… 24
neglect of child (E) …………………………………………………………… 49
néo-Jacksonisme (F) ………………………………………………………… 53
neologism (E) ………………………………………………………………… 28
Nervosität (M. Morita) (D) …………………………………………………… 52
neurasthenia (E) ……………………………………………………………… 53
neuro-Behçet syndrome (disease) (E) ……………………………………… 53
neurodevelopmental hypothesis (E) ………………………………………… 53
neurogenic bladder (E) ……………………………………………………… 52
neuroleptica (L) ……………………………………………………………… 52
neuroleptic-induced acute dystonia (E) …………………………………… 52
neuroleptic-induced akathisia (E) ………………………………………… 52
neuroleptic-induced parkinsonism (E) …………………………………… 52
neuroleptic-induced tardive dyskinesia (E) ……………………………… 52
neuroleptic malignant syndrome (E) ……………………………………… 1, 52
neuroleptics (E) ……………………………………………………………… 52
neurology (E) ………………………………………………………………… 52
neuropathology (E) …………………………………………………………… 53
neuropeptide (E) ……………………………………………………………… 53
neuroplegica (L) ……………………………………………………………… 52
neuropsychiatry (E) …………………………………………………………… 53
neuropsychological examination (E) ………………………………………… 52
neuropsychology (E) ………………………………………………………… 52
neuropsychopharmacology (E) ……………………………………………… 53

neuroscience （E） ……………………………………………………… 52
Neurose （D） …………………………………………………………… 52
neurosis （E） …………………………………………………………… 52
neurosyphilis （E） ……………………………………………………… 72
neurosyphillis （E） ……………………………………………………… 53
Neurosyphillis （D） …………………………………………………… 53
neurotic depression （E） ……………………………………………… 52
neurotic habituation （E） …………………………………………… 52
neurotic overlay （E） ………………………………………………… 52
neurotische Depression （D） ………………………………………… 52
neurotoxin （E） ………………………………………………………… 53
neurotransmitter （E） ………………………………………………… 53
névrose （F） …………………………………………………………… 52
nicotine dependence （DSM-III-R）（E） …………………………… 80
nicotine-related disorder （DSM-IV）（E） ………………………… 80
Niemann-Pick disease （E） ………………………………………… 80
night delirium （E） …………………………………………………… 101
night hospital （E） …………………………………………………… 79
nightmare （E） ………………………………………………………… 1
night terrors （E） ……………………………………………………… 101
nihilistischer Wahn （D） …………………………………………… 24
noatropic drug （E） …………………………………………………… 32
nocturnal drinking syndrome （E） ………………………………… 100
nocturnal eating syndrome （E） …………………………………… 101
nocturnal enuresis （E） ……………………………………………… 100
nocturnal myoclonus （E） …………………………………………… 101
non-24-hour sleep-wake syndrome （E） …………………………… 89
non-attendance at school （E） ……………………………………… 92
non-compliance （E） ………………………………………………… 83
noncompos mentis （E） ……………………………………………… 54
nondominant hemisphere （E） ……………………………………… 105
nonfluent aphasia （E） ……………………………………………… 90
non organic sleep disorder （ICD-10）（E） ………………………… 87
non-REM sleep （E） ………………………………………………… 83

non-verbal communication (E) ……………………………………………… 87
Noopsyche (E. Stransky) (D) ……………………………………………… 71
nootropics (E) ……………………………………………………………… 32
normalization (E) …………………………………………………………… 83
normal pressure hydrocephalus (E) ……………………………………… 57
nosology (E) ………………………………………………………………… 43
nosophobia (E) ……………………………………………………………… 43
nuchal stiffness (E) ………………………………………………………… 32
(nuclear) magnetic resonance spectroscopy (E) ……………………… 9
nuclear ophthalmoplegia (E) …………………………………………… 12
Numinose (R. Otto) (D) ………………………………………………… 81
nursing home (E) ………………………………………………………… 102
nursing home for the aged (E) ………………………………………… 106
nursing home for the aged under poor conditions (E) ……………… 78
nyctophobia (E) …………………………………………………………… 25
nymphomania (E) ……………………………………………………… 50, 81
nystagmus (E) …………………………………………………………… 16
object agnosia (E) ………………………………………………………… 92
object libido (E) …………………………………………………………… 67
object loss (E) ……………………………………………………………… 67
object relations theory (E) ……………………………………………… 67
obligatory symptom (E) ………………………………………………… 88
obnubilation (F) …………………………………………………………… 4
obsession (E) ……………………………………………………………… 23
obsessional ritual (E) …………………………………………………… 23
obsessive-compulsive disorder (E) …………………………………… 23
obsessive idea (E) ………………………………………………………… 23
obsessive slowness (E) ………………………………………………… 23
occasional criminal (E) ………………………………………………… 17
occasional homosexuality (E) ………………………………………… 17
occasional seizures (E) ………………………………………………… 48
occupational delirium (E) ……………………………………………… 36
occupational mental health (E) ………………………………………… 37
occupational problem (E) ……………………………………………… 50

occupational therapist （OT）（E） ……………………………………………… 36
occupational therapy（E） …………………………………………………………… 36
oculogyric crisis（E） …………………………………………………………… 15, 72
Oedipus complex（E） ………………………………………………………………… 9
Ohnmacht（D） ……………………………………………………………………… 42
oily face（E） ………………………………………………………………………… 1
olfactory hallucinatory seizure（E） …………………………………………… 28
olfactory seizure（E） ……………………………………………………………… 20
oligophrenia（E） …………………………………………………………………… 60
oligophrenia phenylpyruvica（L） ……………………………………………… 91
onchophagia（E） …………………………………………………………………… 74
oneiroide Erlebnisform（W. Mayer-Gross）（D） ……………………………… 98
oneiroider Zustand（D） …………………………………………………………… 98
oneirophrenia（L. J. Meduna）（E） ……………………………………………… 98
oniomania（E） …………………………………………………………………… 103
onirisme（E. Régis）（F） ………………………………………………………… 98
only child（E） ……………………………………………………………………… 88
onomatomania（E） ………………………………………………………………… 98
onomatopoeia（E） ………………………………………………………………… 17
open door system（E） …………………………………………………………… 90
operant conditioning（E） …………………………………………………………… 9
operation diagnosis（E） ………………………………………………………… 65
ophthalmoplegia（E） ……………………………………………………………… 15
opioid（DSM-IV）（E） ……………………………………………………………… 1
opioid abuse（E） …………………………………………………………………… 2
opioid dependence（E） …………………………………………………………… 1
opioid-induced（DSM-IV）（E） …………………………………………………… 2
opioid-induced disorder（E） ……………………………………………………… 2
opioid-induced mood disorders（E） …………………………………………… 2
opioid-induced psychotic disorder（E） ………………………………………… 2
opioid-induced sexual dysfunction（E） ………………………………………… 2
opioid-induced sleep disorders（E） …………………………………………… 2
opioid intoxication（E） …………………………………………………………… 1
opioid intoxication delirium（E） ………………………………………………… 1

opioid-related disorders (DSM-IV) (E) 1
opioid use disorders (E) 1
opioid withdrawal (E) 2
opisthotonus (E) 102
oppositional defiant disorder (DSM-IV) (E) 86
optic ataxia (E) 37
optische Ataxie (M. Balint) (D) 37
optokinetic nystagmus (OKN) (E) 37
oral character (E) 30
oral dyskinesia (E) 32
orality (E) 30
Oral-Petit mal (D. Janz) (D) 32
oral phase (E) 30
oral tendency (E) 25
organ erotism (E) 17
organic (E) 18, 20
organic amnesic syndrome (ICD-10) (E) 18
organic anxiety disorder (ICD-10) (E) 18
organic bipolar affective disorder (ICD-10) (E) 18
organic catatonic disorder (ICD-10) (E) 18
organic delusional (schizophrenia-like) disorder (ICD-10) (E) 18
organic delusional state (E) 18
organic dementia (E) 18
organic depressive disorder (E) 18
organic dissociative disorder (E) 18
organic emotionally labile (asthenic) disorder (ICD-10) (E) 18
organic hallucinosis (ICD-10) (E) 18
organic manic disorder (ICD-10) (E) 18
organic mental disorder (ICD-10) (E) 18
organic mixed affective disorder (ICD-10) (E) 18
organic mood (affective) disorder (ICD-10) (E) 18
organic personality disorder (ICD-10) (E) 18
organic psychosis (E) 18
organic solvent abuse (E) 101

organ inferiority（E）	17
organisches Psychosyndrom（E. Bleuler）（D）	18
organisches Psychosyndrom（M. Bleuler）（D）	82
organization of the family with the mentally ill（E）	13
organ language（E）	17
Organminderwertigkeit（A. Adler）（D）	17
Organneurose（D）	17
organodynamisme（H. Ey）（F）	18
Organwahl（D）	17
orgasmic dysfunction（E）	10
orientation（E）	29
Orientierung（D）	29
orthochromatic leukodystrophy（E）	61
orthopsychiatry（E）	22
örtliche Desorientiertheit（D）	84
Othello syndrome（J. Todd & K. Dewhurst）（E）	9
outpatient（E）	6, 11
overadjustment（E）	13
overanxious disorder of child（E）	49
overcompensation（E）	13
overvalue idea（E）	44
pain disorder（DSM-IV）（E）	77
palatal myoclonus（E）	30
paligraphia（E）	50
palilalia（E）	77
palliative care（E）	17
palliative care unit（E）	17
palliative medicine（E）	17
palmomental reflex（E）	46
panic attack（DSM-III）（E）	85
panic disorder（ICD-10, DSM-III-R）（E）	85
papillary stasis（E）	7
papilledema（E）	7
parabulia（E）	6

paradoxical reaction (E)	17
paradoxical sleep (E)	20
paragrammatism (E)	36
paragraphia (E)	36
paralexia (E)	36
paralipophobia (E)	95
paralogia (E)	36
paralysis agitans (L)	54
paralytic attack (E)	96
paramnesia (E)	17
paranoia (E)	85
paranoid personality disorder (ICD-9, DSM-III) (E)	99
paranoid reaction (E)	100
paranoid-schizoid position (E)	85
paranoid schizophrenia (E)	99
paranoid state (E)	99
paraphasia (E)	36
paraphilia (E)	85
paraphrenia (E)	85
paraplegia in extension (E)	55
paraplegia in flexion (E)	25
parapraxia (E)	36
parasomnia (E)	56, 85
parataxic distortion (H. S. Sullivan) (E)	85
parathymia (E)	20
paratonia (E)	85
paratonic rigidity (E)	74
paratony (E)	85
pareidoria (E)	85
parens patriae power (E)	25
paresthesia (E)	36
pariomania (E)	83
Parkinson-dementia complex (E)	84
Parkinson disease (E)	84

Parkinsonian syndrome (E) ……………………………………………………… 83
Parkinsonism (E) ………………………………………………………………… 83
Parkinsonism-dementia complex (E) ………………………………………… 84
paroxysmal dysrhythmia (E) …………………………………………………… 78
parrot-like speaking (E) ………………………………………………………… 9
partial agonist (E) ………………………………………………………………… 84
partial amnesia (E) ……………………………………………………………… 92
partial epilepsy (E) ……………………………………………………………… 92
partial hospitalization (E) ……………………………………………………… 92
partialism (E) …………………………………………………………………… 92
partial object relationship (E) ………………………………………………… 92
partial seizure (E) ……………………………………………………………… 92
participant observation (H. S. Sullivan) (E) ……………………………… 16
passive-aggressive personality disorder (DSM-III) (E) ………………… 47
passivité (F) …………………………………………………………………… 88
past-pointing test (E) ………………………………………………………… 40
paternalism (E) ………………………………………………………………… 84
pathogenetisch (K. Birnbaum) (D) ………………………………………… 89
Pathographie (D) ……………………………………………………………… 89
pathography (E) ………………………………………………………………… 89
pathological gambling (E) …………………………………………………… 90
pathological lying (E) ………………………………………………………… 90
pathologischer Rausch (D) …………………………………………………… 90
pathologischer Schwindler (D) ……………………………………………… 89
pathophobia (E) ………………………………………………………………… 43
pathoplastisch (K. Birnbaum) (D) …………………………………………… 89
patient club (E) ………………………………………………………………… 15
patient council (E) ……………………………………………………………… 15
patient government (E) ……………………………………………………… 15
pavor nocturnus (L) …………………………………………………………… 101
pedophilia (E) …………………………………………………………………… 49
pellagra psychosis (E) ………………………………………………………… 94
Pensionsneurose (D) ………………………………………………………… 81
perceive reality as it is (E) …………………………………………………… 2

perceptual alteration (E)	71
perceptual rivalry (E)	70
perfect remission (E)	16
performance intelligence quotient (PIQ) (E)	77
periodic limb movement disorder (E)	45
periodic psychosis (E)	45
periodic somnolence (E)	45
periodic synchronous discharge (PSD) (E)	45
periodische Schlafsucht (D)	45
periodische Verstimmung (D)	45
period of opposition (E)	85
perplexity (E)	35
persécuté persécuteur (F)	12
perseveration (E)	95
persistent (E)	20
persistent delusional disorders (E)	41
persistent insomnia (E)	41
personality (E)	84
personality change (E)	52
personality disorder (ICD-9, DSM-III) (E)	51
personality disorder cluster A (DSM-III-R) (E)	8
Personenverkennung (D)	55
personification (E)	19
Persönlichkeitsniveausenkung (D)	51
Persönlichkeitsreaktion (D)	52
Persönlichkeitsveränderung (D)	52, 56
Persönlichkeitszerfall (D)	52
personnalité pathologique (F)	51
person responsible for protection (E)	95
person responsible for support (E)	92
persuasion therapy (E)	63
pervasive developmental disorders (DSM-III) (E)	32
petit mal (F)	49
petit mal absence (E)	49

petit mal status （E） ……………………………………………………… 49
petit mal variant （F. A .& E. L. Gibbs）（E） ……………………… 49
petit mal variant absence （E） ………………………………………… 49
phallic stage （E） ………………………………………………………… 70
Phäneomenologie （D） ………………………………………………… 29
phänomenologische Psychopathologie （D） ………………………… 29
phantastic confabulation （E） ………………………………………… 25
phantom boarder （E） ………………………………………………… 96
Phantomglied （D） ……………………………………………………… 28
phantom limb （E） ……………………………………………………… 28
pharmacotherapy （E） ………………………………………………… 101
pharyngeal reflex （E） ………………………………………………… 7
phase （E） ………………………………………………………………… 89
Phase （D） ………………………………………………………………… 89
phénomène xénopatique （P. Guiraud）（F） ………………………… 11
phénoménologie （F） …………………………………………………… 29
phenomenology （E） …………………………………………………… 29
phenotype （E） …………………………………………………………… 89
phenylketonuria （E） …………………………………………………… 90
phobia （E） ……………………………………………………………… 23
phobic anxiety disorder （ICD-10）（E） …………………………… 23
phonemic paraphasia （E） …………………………………………… 10
phonological disorder （DSM-Ⅳ）（E） …………………………… 10
photic synesthesia （E） ………………………………………………… 22
photism （E） ……………………………………………………………… 22
photogenic epilepsy （E） ……………………………………………… 30
photoma （E） …………………………………………………………… 102
photosensitive epilepsy （E） ………………………………………… 87
phototherapy （E） ……………………………………………………… 31
phrenology （E） ………………………………………………………… 34
physical abuse （E） …………………………………………………… 54
physical dependence （E） …………………………………………… 54
physical therapy （treatment）（E） ………………………………… 55
physikalischer Beeinträchtigungswahn （D） ……………………… 92

Physiognomik (D)	66
pica (L)	5
Pick disease (E)	88
Pickwickian syndrome (E)	88
picture agnosia (E)	13
placebo (E)	93
plasma concentration of drug (E)	101
plasma level of drug (E)	101
Platzangst (D)	90
play therapy (E)	101
pleasure principle (E)	11
pneumoencephalography (E)	19
polygene inheritance (E)	68
polygraph (E)	95
polygraphy (E)	96
polyphagia (E)	69
polysomnography (E)	96
polyspikes (E)	69
polysubstance dependence (DSM-III-R) (E)	69
polysubstance-related disorder (DSM-IV) (E)	69
polysurgery (E)	90
porcupine dilemma (E)	101
porencephaly (E)	32
positional vertigo (E)	75
Positive and Negative Syndrome Scale (PANSS) (E)	102
positive symptom (E)	102
positron emission tomography (PET) (E)	95
possession (E)	89
postconcussion syndrome (ICD-10) (E)	82
posterior aphasia (E)	32
post-hypnotic suggestion (E)	36
postictal automatism (E)	95
postictal psychosis (E)	95
postoperative psychosis (E)	46

postpartum depression（E） ……………………………………………………… 37
postpsychotic depression（E） ………………………………………………… 61
postschizophrenic depression（E） …………………………………………… 76
poststroke depression（E） …………………………………………………… 82
post-traumatic stress disorder（PTSD）（E） ………………………………… 55
postural reflex（E） …………………………………………………………… 41
postural seizure（E） ………………………………………………………… 41
postural tremor（E） ………………………………………………………… 41
postural vertigo（E） ………………………………………………………… 41
Prader-Willi syndrome（E） …………………………………………………… 93
Praecoxgefühl（H. C. Rümke）（D） ………………………………………… 93
precipitating factor（E） ……………………………………………………… 27
preconscious（E） ……………………………………………………………… 63
predisposition（E） …………………………………………………………… 65
predominantly hyperactive-impulsive type（E） ……………………………… 72
predominantly inattentive type（E） ………………………………………… 72
prefrontal leucotomy（E. Moniz）（E） ……………………………………… 65
pregenital stage（E） ………………………………………………………… 64
prematura sexualis（L） ……………………………………………………… 62
premature ejaculation（E） …………………………………………………… 66
premenstrual tension syndrome（R. T. Frank）（E） ………………………… 27
premorbid personality（E） …………………………………………………… 89
prepsychotic stage（E） ……………………………………………………… 64
presbyophrenia（E） …………………………………………………………… 93
Presbyophrenie（D） …………………………………………………………… 93
presenile dementia（E） ……………………………………………………… 50
present state examination（PSE）（E） ……………………………………… 28
preterm infant（E） …………………………………………………………… 65
prevalence（E） ……………………………………………………………… 102
preventive psychiatry（E） ………………………………………………… 103
primärer Wahn（D） …………………………………………………………… 5
primary care（E） …………………………………………………………… 92
primary delusion（E） ………………………………………………………… 5
primary drive（E） …………………………………………………………… 5

primary epilepsy (E) 29
primary gain (E) 5
primary scene (E) 28
priming (E) 92
primitive defence mechanism (E) 29
primitive idealization (E) 29
primitive reaction (E) 29
prison psychosis (E) 30
prison reaction (E) 30
proband (E) 95
probationary supervision (E) 95
procedural memory (E) 74
prodromal schizophrenia (E) 63
prodromal state (E) 63
profound mental retardation (E) 35, 60
progressive multifocal leukoencephalopathy (PML) (E) 53
progressive Paralyse (D) 53
progressive supranuclear palsy (PSP) (E) 53
projection (E) 76
projective identification (M. Klein) (E) 75
projective method (E) 76
Projektion (D) 76
prolonged depression (E) 63
Propfschizophrenie (D) 63
Propfhebephrenie (D) 63
Propulsiv-Petit mal (D. Janz) (D) 63
prosopagnosia (E) 66
protopathic sensation (E) 28
Protreptik (D) 26
provozierte Depression (J. Lange) (D) 102
pseudobulbar palsy (paralysis) (E) 13
pseudodementia (E) 13
pseudohallucination (E) (F) 13
pseudologia phantastica (L) 25

pseudomnesia (E)	13
pseudomutuality (L. Wynne) (E)	19
pseudoneurotic schizophrenia (E)	19
psychagogics (E)	21
psychalgia (E)	60
psychasthénie (P. Janet) (F)	60
psychiatric bed (E)	58
psychiatric demography (E)	57
psychiatric drug therapy (E)	58
psychiatric epidemiology (E)	57
psychiatric evidence (E)	58
psychiatric expertise before indictment (E)	19
psychiatric nursing (E)	58
psychiatric occupational therapy (E)	58
psychiatric rehabilitation (E)	58
psychiatric review board (E)	57
psychiatric social worker (PSW) (E)	61
psychiatric testimony (E)	58
psychiatric visiting nursing (E)	58
psychiatrie medico-légale (F)	44
psychiatrische Begutachtung (D)	58
psychiatrisches Gutachten (D)	58
psychiatrist (E)	58
psychiatry (E)	57
psychical seizure (W. Penfield) (E)	61
psychic dependence (E)	57
psychic determinism (E)	55
psychic energizer (E)	61
psychic energy (E)	55
psychic gaze paralysis (E)	60
psychic interaction (E)	58
psychic seizure (W. G. Lennox) (E)	61
psychic trauma (E)	55
Psychiker (D)	61

psychoactive substance（ICD-10）（E） ……………………………………… 58
psychoanalysis（E） ……………………………………………………………… 61
psychobiology（A. Meyer）（E） ……………………………………………… 60
psychodrama（E） ………………………………………………………………… 35
psychodrama（J. L. Moreno）（E） …………………………………………… 55
psychodynamics（E） …………………………………………………………… 61
psychoeducation（E） …………………………………………………………… 55
psychogene Überlagerung（D） ……………………………………………… 51
psychogenic（E） ………………………………………………………………… 51
psychogenic amnesia（E） ……………………………………………………… 51
psychogenic depression（E） ………………………………………………… 51
psychogenic fugue（E） ………………………………………………………… 51
psychogenic overlay（E） ……………………………………………………… 51
psychogenic polydipsia（E） …………………………………………………… 51
psychogenic psychosis（E） …………………………………………………… 51
psychogenic reaction（E） ……………………………………………………… 51
psychogenic stupor（E） ………………………………………………………… 51
psychogenic vomiting（E） ……………………………………………………… 51
Psychogenie（R. Sommer）（D） ……………………………………………… 51
psychoimmunology（E） ………………………………………………………… 61
psychological testing（E） ……………………………………………………… 55
psychologie en profondeur（F） ……………………………………………… 54
psychometry（E） ……………………………………………………………… 55, 60
Psychomotorik（D） ……………………………………………………………… 57
psychomotorische Hemmung（D） …………………………………………… 57
psychomotorishe Erregung（D） ……………………………………………… 57
psychomotor seizure（E） ……………………………………………………… 57
psychonephrology（E） ………………………………………………………… 35
psychoneuroimmunology（E） ………………………………………………… 60
psychoneurosis（E） ……………………………………………………………… 60
psychooncology（E） …………………………………………………………… 35
psychopathische Persönlichkeit（K. Schneider）（D） ……………………… 61
Psychopathologie（D） ………………………………………………………… 61
psychopathology（E） …………………………………………………………… 61

psychopharmacology（E）	61
psychophysiological insomnia（E）	60
psychophysiology（E）	60
Psychose（D）	61
psychose（F）	61
psychose hallucinatoire chronique（G. Ballet）（F）	96
psychose maniaco-dépressive（F）	65
psychose passionnelle（G. G. de Clérambault）（F）	81
psychose polynervritique（F）	69
psychosis（E）	61
psychosomatic correlation（E）	53
psychosomatic disease（E）	53
psychosomatic medicine（E）	53
psychosomatische Krankheit（D）	53
psychostimulant（E）	59, 72
psychosurgery（E）	58
psychotherapy（E）	61
psychotropic drug（E）	31
pubertas praecox（L）	62
Pubertätskrise（D）	40
Pubertätsmagersucht（D）	40
Pubertätsparanoia（D）	40
Public Assistance Law（E）	57
puerilism（E）	102
puerperal depression（E）	37
puerperal mental disorders（E）	37
puerperal psychosis（E）	37
pulsion（F）	103
punch-drunk syndrome（E）	95
pure agraphia（E）	47
pure alexia（E）	47
pure amnesia（E）	47
pure petit mal（E）	47
pure word-deafness（E）	47

pure word-dumbness （E） 47
pursuit of thinness （E） 101
pyknic （E） 92
Pykniker （D） 92
pyknolepsy （E） 87
pyromania （E） 94
quadrantanopsia （E） 44
quality of life （QOL）（E） 57
quasi-incompetence （E） 89
Querulant （D） 31
Querulantenwahn （D） 32
querulous delusion （E） 32
questionnaire method （E） 43
rabbit syndrome （E） 103
railway spine （E） 74
Randneurose （J. H. Schultz）（D） 94
randomized clinical trial （RCT）（E） 98
Randsymptom （D） 94
rapid cycler （E） 103
rapid eye movement （E） 21
rapport （F） 103
raptus melancholicus （L） 99
rating scale for the assesement of psychiatric symptom （E） 60
rational emotive therapy （E） 106
rationales Verstehen （D） 33
rationalisme morbide （E. Minkowski）（F） 90
rationalization （E） 32
Ratlosigkeit （D） 35
Raumerleben （D） 25
Rausch （D） 99
reaction formation （E） 86
reactive amnesia （E） 86
reactive attachment disorder （E） 86
reactive depression （E） 86

reactive excitement（E）	86
reactive psychosis（E）	86
reading disorder（ICD-10, DSM-Ⅲ）（E）	78
reading epilepsy（E）	78
reading retardation（ICD-9）（E）	78
Reaktionsbildung（D）	86
Realangst（S. Freud）（D）	29
Realitätsprinzip（D）	28
Realitätsprüfung（D）	28
Realitätsbewußtsein（D）	28
reality orientation（E）	28
reality principle（E）	28
reality testing（E）	28
rebound insomnia（E）	86
recent memory（E）	24
receptive aphasia（E）	47
receptive language disorder（ICD-10）（E）	47
receptor（E）	47
recessive（nondoninant）cerebral hemisphere（E）	105
Rechtslinksstörung（D）	37
recognition（E）	35
recovered memory（E）	11
recreational therapy（E）	105
recurrence（E）	35
recurrent（E）	20
recurrent depressive disorder（ICD-10）（E）	86
recurrent hypersomnia（E）	86
Rededrang（D）	70
Reduktion des energetischen Potentials（K. Conrad）（D）	9
reduplicating paramnesia（E）	73
reduplicative paramnesia（E）	46
reduplizierende Paramnesie（A. Pick）（D）	46
reference upon one's own self（E）	40
reflex epilepsy（E）	86

R

reflex hallucination (E)	86
refoulement (F)	102
reframing (E)	104
regression (E)	67
rehabilitaiton (E)	104
reiner Defekt (G. Huber) (D)	47
reizbare Schwäche (D)	39
Reizbarkeit (D)	5, 39
relapse (E)	35
religious delusion (E)	45
remedial education (E)	73
remission (E)	14
Remission (D)	14
REM latency (E)	105
remote memory (E)	9
REM (rapid eye movement) sleep (E)	105
REM sleep behavior disorder (E)	105
Rentenneurose (D)	83
reparation (M. Klein) (E)	74
repetition-compulsion (E)	86
repression (E)	102
répression (F)	103
reproduction (E)	35
Reproduktion (D)	35
residual epilepsy (E)	37
residual schizophrenia (E)	37
Residualwahn (D)	37
resistance analysis (E)	74
respiratory affect spasm (E)	93
resting tremor (E)	57
restless legs syndrome (E)	13
rest word (E)	37
retention (E)	95
retrograde amnesia (E)	20

Retropulsiv-petit-mal (D. Janz) (D) ... 30
Rett syndrome (disorder) (E) ... 105
revenge enuresis (E) ... 91
reverse tolerance phenomenon (E) ... 20
reversible dementia (E) ... 12
revolving door phenomenon (E) ... 11
reward system (E) ... 94
Reye syndrome (E) ... 103
Rezidiv (D) ... 35
rhythmic movement disorder (E) ... 104
righting reflex (E) ... 69
right-left disorientation (E) ... 37
right of treatment (E) ... 73
right to refuse treatment (E) ... 73
rigidity (E) ... 33
Rindenblindheit (D) ... 88
ripple wave (E) ... 105
Rorschach test (E) ... 106
Rosenzweig Picture-Frustration Study (E) ... 87
rotatory vertigo (E) ... 11
rumination disorder (DSM-III) (E) ... 86
rumination mentale (P. Janet) (F) ... 55
sadism (E) ... 12
Salbengesicht (D) ... 1
Sammelsucht (D) ... 45
sand play (E) ... 84
Sandspiel (D) ... 84
satyriasis (E) ... 36, 70
Scale for the Assessment of Negative Symptoms (SANS) (E) ... 7
scanning speech (E) ... 70
scène originaire (F) ... 28
Schauanfall (D) ... 72
Schaulust (D) ... 63
Schichtdiagnose (D) ... 66

Schichtentheorie (D)	66
Schichtneurose (J. H. Schultz) (D)	65
Schicksalsanalyse (L. Szondi) (D)	8
Schicksalszwang (S. Freud) (D)	8
Schilder disease (E)	51
schizo-affective disorder (ICD-10, DSM-III) (E)	76
schizo-affective psychosis (J. Kassanin) (E)	76
schizoid (E)	76
schizoid personality disorder (ICD-10, DSM-III) (E)	76
schizomanie (H. Claude) (F)	105
schizophasia (E)	76
schizophrenia (E)	58, 61, 70, 76
schizophrenia hebephrenic type (E)	83
schizophrenia paranoid type (E)	99
schizophrenic dementia (E)	76
schizophrenic reaction (E)	76
Schizophrenie (D)	76
schizophreniform disorder (DSM-III) (E)	77
schizophreniform psychosis (G. Langfeldt) (E)	77
schizophrenogenic mother (F. Fromm-Reichmann) (E)	77
schizothymia (E)	76
schizotypal disorder (ICD-10) (E)	76
schizotypal personality disorder (DSM-III) (E)	76
Schlafanfall (D)	56
Schlafepilepsie (D. Janz) (D)	56
Schlafsucht (D)	44
Schlaftrunkenheit (D)	81
Schlafwandeln (D)	98
Schlafzeremonie (D)	46
Schlüsselerlebnis (E. Kretschmer) (D)	12
Schmerzasymbolie (D)	74
Schnauzkrampf (D)	78
school for the handicapped (E)	102
school phobia (E)	14

school refusal (E)	76
school truancy (E)	67
Schreckepilepsie (D)	22
Schreckreaktion (D)	22
Schreibkrampf (D)	50
Schub (D)	47
Schuldfähigkeit (D)	62
Schuldgefühl (D)	35
Schuldunfähigkeit (D)	62
Schwachsinn (D)	60
Schwangerschaftspsychose (D)	81
Schwerbesinnlichkeit (D)	98
scintillating scotoma (E)	63
scissors gait (E)	84
screen memory (E)	7
seasonal affective disorder (E)	15, 19
seasonal depression (E)	19
secondary delusion (E)	80
secondary epilepsy (E)	66
secondary gain (E)	79
second generation antipsychotics (SGA) (E)	68
Seelenblindheit (D)	61
Seelenheilkunde (D)	60
Seelenlähmung des Schauens (D)	60
Seelentaubheit (D)	61
segmental apraxia (E)	93
seizure (E)	95
seizure discharge (E)	95
seizure with impairment of consciousness (E)	4
sekundärer Wahn (D)	79
Selbstbewußtsein (D)	39
Selbsterhaltungstrieb (D)	40
Selbstgespräch (D)	78
Selbstmord (D)	40

Selbstmordgedanke (D) 40
Selbstmordversuch (D) 40
Selbstreflexion (D) 79
Selbstschilderung (D) 40
Selbstunsichere (Psychopathen) (K. Schneider) (D) 41
Selbstverletzung (D) 41
Selbstverstümmelung (D) 41
Selbstvorwurf (D) 41
selective amnesia (E) 64
selective inattention (H. S. Sullivan) (E) 64
selective mutism (E) 64
selective serotonin reuptake inhibitor (SSRI) (E) 64
self-accusation (E) 41
self-centered (E) 40
self consciousness (E) 39
self-directed (E) 40
self-help group (E) 41
self-mutilation (E) 41
semantic amnesia (E) 6
semantic aphasia (E) 33
semantic memory (E) 6
senile dementia (E) 106
senile dementia of Alzheimer type (SDAT) (E) 3
senile dementia with neurofibrillary tangle (SD-NFT) (E) 52
senile psychosis (E) 106
sensitiver Beziehungswahn (E. Kretschmer) (D) 90
Sensitivparanoia (D) 90
sensorium (E) 38
sensory aphasia (E) 14
sensory deprivation (E) 14
sensory dissociation (E) 14
sensory distortion (E) 71
sensory extinction (E) 14
sensory memory (E) 14

sentence completion test（SCT）（E）	93
sentiment（F）	15
sentiment（E）	48
sentiment d'appropriation au moi（F）	40
sentiment d'influence（F）	87
sentiment d'irréel（F）	87
sentiment du vide（P. Janet）（F）	25
separation anxiety（E）	93
separation anxiety disorder（E）	93
separation-individuation（E）	93
serotonin-dopamine inhibitor（E）	63
serotonin-noradrenaline reuptake inhibitor（SNRI）（E）	63
services and supports for persons with disabilities act（E）	47
severe mental retardation（E）	46, 60
severeness of school attendance（E）	92
sexual abuse（E）	61
sexual abuse of child（E）	49
sexual arousal disorder（E）	62
sexual aversion disorder（E）	57
sexual dysfunction（E）	57
sexual frigidity（E）	62
sexual harassment（E）	63
sexual masochism（E）	62
sexual neurasthenia（E）	62
sexual pain disorders（E）	57
sexual perversion（E）	62
sexual sadism（E）	62
shamanism（E）	45
shared psychotic disorder（DSM-IV-TR）（E）	23
sharp wave（E）	8
shell shock（E）	95
sheltered work institution for mentally handicapped person（E）	46
sheltered work institution for the person with mental disorder（E）	59
sheltered workshop（E）	95

Shinkeishitsu（森田正馬）（J）	52
short circuit reaction（E）	70
short sleeper（E）	70
short term memory（E）	70
short-term psychotherapy（E）	70
Shy-Drager syndrome（E）	44
sibling rivalry（E）	77
sibling rivalry disorder（ICD-10）（E）	78
Sicherungsmaßnahme（D）	94
Silbenstolpern（D）	74
simple deteriorative disorder（E）	70
simple drunkenness（E）	70
simple schizophrenia（E）	70
simple type（E）	70
simulation（E）	37
Simulation（D）	37
simultanagnosia（E）	77
Simultanagnosie（D）	77
single photon emission computed tomography（SPECT）（E）	70
Sinnesgedächtnis（D）	14
Sinnestäuschung（D）	14
sitiophobia（E）	50
Situagenie（D）	47
situational mutism（E）	85
situational reaction（E）	15
situation-related seizure（E）	48
situative Desorientierung（D）	48
sleep apnea syndrome（E）	56
sleep attack（E）	56
sleep deprivation（E）	70
sleep disorder（E）	56
sleep disturbance of shift worker（E）	32
sleep paralysis（E）	56
sleep terror disorder（E）	56

sleep-wake schedule disorder（E）	56
sleep walking（E）	98
sleepwalking disorder（ICD-10）（E）	56
slow burst（E）	50
slowly progressive aphasia（E）	16
slow wave（E）	50
snout reflex（E）	25
social adaptation training for the person with mental disorder（E）	59
social and occupational functioning assessment scale（E）	44
social anxiety disorder（DSM-IV）（E）	45
social brain（E）	44
socialization（E）	44
social pathology（E）	44
social phobia（DSM-III）（E）	45
social psychiatry（E）	44
social readjustment rating scale（E）	44
social rehabilitation facility for the person with mental disorder（E）	59
social remission（E）	44
social skills training（SST）（E）	44
social welfare（E）	45
sociogenic（E）	44
sociometry（J. L. Moreno）（E）	44
Sodomie（D）	45
sodomy（E）	32
somatic symptoms（E）	54
Somatiker（D）	55
Somatisierung（D）	54
somatization（E）	54
somatization disorder（E）	54
somatoform disorder（E）	55
somatogenic（E）	66
somatognostic disorder（E）	55
Somatopsyche（C. Wernicke）（D）	54
somnambulism（E）	98

S

somnolence (E)	26
Somnolenz (D)	26
soporifics (E)	56
source amnesia (E)	46
souvenir traumatique (F)	11
soziale Remission (D)	44
space phobia (E)	25
spasm (E)	26
spastic gait (E)	26
spasticity (E)	26
spastic paralysis (E)	26
Spätdepression (D)	71
Spätepilepsie (D)	71
spatial disorientation (E)	83
Spätkatatonie (M. Sommer) (D)	71
Spätschizophrenie (D)	71
special education (E)	78
specific developmental disorder (ICD-10, DSM-III) (E)	78
specific developmental disorder of motor function (ICD-10) (E)	8
specific developmental disorders of scholastic skills (ICD-10 新訂版) (E)	12
specific developmental disorders of speech and language (ICD-10) (E)	12
specific disorder of arithmetical skills (ICD-10) (E)	78
specific reading disorder (ICD-10) (E)	78
specific speech articulation disorder (ICD-10) (E)	77
specific spelling disorder (ICD-10) (E)	78
speech center (E)	28
Sperrung (D)	78
spike (E)	24
spike-and-wave complex (E)	24
spike-wave stupor (E)	24
spindle (E)	95
splitting (E)	56
Spontaneitätsmangel (D)	44
Spontansprechen (D)	44

Sprachstereotypie (D)	28
Sprachverwirrtheit (D)	28
stade du miroir (J. Lacan) (F)	22
stand alone (E)	88
startle epilepsy (E)	22
startle reaction (E)	22
stationäre Paralyse (D)	74
stationary paresis (E)	74
statisches Verstehen (D)	62
status epilepticus (L)	75
Stauungspapille (D)	7
stehende Redensart (D)	68
Stehltrieb (D)	77
steppage gait (E)	26
stereotype/habit disorder (E)	48
stereotype movement disorder (E)	48
stereotypy (E)	49
steroid psychosis (E)	56
sthenisch (D)	23
stiffness (E)	33
stigma (E)	56
Stimmenhören (D)	29
Stimmungslabile (Psychopathen) (K. Schneider) (D)	20
Stimmungslabilität (D)	19
Stirnhirnsyndrom (D)	65
stormy personality (S. Arieti) (E)	56
Stottern (D)	19
Straffähigkeit (D)	46
stranger anxiety (E)	88
stranger reaction (E)	88
stratification theory (E)	66
stress (E)	56
stressor (E)	56
striatonigral degeneration (SND) (E)	64

structural interview (E)	31
structured interview (E)	31
structure of psychotherapy (E)	73
Strukturanalyse (K. Birnbaum) (D)	31
student apathy (E)	12
Stupor (D)	35
stupor (E)	35
Sturge-Weber disease (E)	56
stuttering (E)	19
subacute necrotizing encephalo-myelopathy (Leigh disease) (E)	1
subacute sclerosing panencephalitis (SSPE) (E)	1
subacute spongiform encephalopathy (SSE) (E)	1
subcortical aphasia (E)	87
subcortical dementia (E)	87
Subdepression (D)	26
sublimation (E)	47
subordinate (cerebral) hemisphere (E)	104
substance abuse (DSM-IV) (E)	59
substance dependence (DSM-IV) (E)	58
substance-induced (E)	20
substance-induced anxiety disorder (E)	59
substance-induced delirium (E)	59
substance-induced disorders (DSM-IV-TR) (E)	59
substance-induced mood disorder (E)	59
substance-induced persisting amnestic disorder (E)	59
substance-induced persisting dementia (E)	59
substance-induced psychotic disorder (E)	59
substance-induced sexual dysfunction (E)	59
substance-induced sleep disorder (E)	59
substance intoxication (DSM-IV) (E)	58
substance intoxication delirium (E)	58
substance-related disorders (DSM-IV) (E)	58
substance use disorders (DSM-III) (E)	58
substance withdrawal (DSM-IV) (E)	59

substance withdrawal delirium （E）	59
substitution （E）	68
substitutive formation （E）	68
Substupor （D）	1
Sucht （D）	44
sucking reflex （E）	20
suggestibility （E）	87
suggestion （E，F）	3
suggestive therapy （E）	3
suicide （E）	40
suicide cluster （E）	25
suicide idea （E）	18
Suizid （D）	40
Sündenwahn （D）	35
sundowner syndrome （E）	101
sundowning syndrome （E）	101
super-ego （E）	73
supervision （E）	56
support （E）	40
support institusion for intellectually disorder （E）	71
supportive psychotherapy （E）	40
suppression （E）	103
supranuclear ophthalmoplegia （E）	12
sustained release dosage form of antipsychotics （E）	39
Sydenham chorea （E）	43
symbiotic infantile psychosis （M. Mahler） （E）	22
symbolization （E）	48
sympathetic apraxia （E）	30
sympathy （E）	22
symptomarme Schizophrenie （D）	13
symptomatic （E）	48
symptomatic epilepsy （E）	48
symptomatic psychosis （E）	48
symptomatic schizophrenia （E）	48

Symptome 1. Ranges（K. Schneider）（D） ············· 5
synapse（E） ············· 43
synchronicity（C. G. Jung）（E） ············· 22
synchronous（E） ············· 76
synchrony（E） ············· 75
syncope（E） ············· 42
syndrome de Cotard（J. Cotard）（F） ············· 34
syndrome d'influence（A. Ceillier）（F） ············· 87
syndrome malin（F） ············· 1
synesthesia（E） ············· 22
Synton（D） ············· 77
syntone（E） ············· 77
synucleinopathy（E） ············· 43
syphilophobia（E） ············· 83
systematic desensitization（E） ············· 26
systematischer Wahn（D） ············· 67
systematized delusion（E） ············· 67
Szondi test（E） ············· 66
Taboparalyse（D） ············· 62
taboparalysis（E） ············· 62
taboparesis（E） ············· 62
tactile agnosia（E） ············· 50
tactile aphasia（E） ············· 50
tactile extinction（E） ············· 50
tactile hallucination（E） ············· 29
Tagesschwankung（D） ············· 80
Tagtraum（D） ············· 84
Tanaka-Binet test（E） ············· 69
tandem gait（E） ············· 74
taphephobia（E） ············· 96
tardive dyskinesia（E） ············· 71
Tatendrang（D） ············· 30
tauopathy（E） ············· 68
tau protein（E） ············· 68

technostress（E）	74
telepathy（E）	75
temperament（E）	18
temperance society（E）	70
temper tantrum（L）	15
temporal disorientation（E）	38
temporal lobe epilepsy（E）	66
tension headache（E）	24
tension psychologique（P. Janet）（F）	55
terminal care（E）	69
terminal sleep（E）	46
test of aphasia（E）	42
tetraplegia（E）	40
tetratogenicity（E）	35
thalamic dementia（E）	41
The Confinement and Protection for Lunatics Act（E）	61
thematic apperception test（TAT）（E）	10
theory of cerebral localization（E）	68
theory of mind（E）	33
therapeutic alliance（E）	73
therapeutic community（E）	73
therapeutic contract（E）	73
therapeutic regression（E）	73
thought broadcasting（E）	31
thought disorder（E）	39
thought echo（E）	31
thought insertion（E）	31
thought withdrawal（E）	31
thumb sucking（E）	9, 102
thymoleptica（L）	15
thyreogenic psychosis（E）	31
tic（E）	71
tic disorder（ICD-10, DSM-III）（E）	71
tic facial（F）	16

Tiefenpsychologie（D）	54
Tierverwandlungswahn（D）	45
time-limited psychotherapy（E）	38
tobacco dependance（DSM-Ⅲ）（E）	69
tödliche Katatonie（K. H. Stauder）（D）	71
toilet training（E）	83
tolerance（E）	67
tonic clonic convulsion（E）	22
tonic clonic seizure（E）	22
tonic convulsion（E）	23
tonic neck reflex（E）	24
tonic seizure（E）	23
tonischer Krampf（D）	23
topographical dysmnesia（E）	71
total amnesia（E）	63
total aphasia（E）	64
Totstellreflex（D）	41
Tourette syndrome（E）	78
toxoplasmosis（E）	78
training therapy（E）	25
traitment moral（F）	100
trance（E）	79
tranquilizer（E）	57
transactional analysis（E. Berne）（E）	33
transcortical aphasia（E）	73
transcortical motor aphasia（E）	73
transcortical sensory aphasia（E）	73
transcranial magnetic stimulation（TMS）（E）	26
transcultural psychiatry（E）	69, 87
transference（E）	75
transfert（F）	75
transient global amnesia（E）	5
transient ischemic attack（TIA）（E）	5
transitional facility（E）	72

transitional object（E） ……………………………………………………………… 4
transitivism（E） ………………………………………………………………… 48
transit syndrome（E） …………………………………………………………… 74
transkortikale Aphasie（D） …………………………………………………… 73
transmissible dementia（E） …………………………………………………… 75
transsexualism（E） ……………………………………………………………… 62
transvestism（E） ………………………………………………………………… 91
transzendentale Phänomenologie（E. Husserl）（D） ……………………… 73
Trauerarbeit（D） ………………………………………………………………… 87
traumatic dementia（E） ………………………………………………………… 11
traumatic epilepsy（E） ………………………………………………………… 11
traumatic memory（E） ………………………………………………………… 11
traumatic neurosis（E） ………………………………………………………… 10
traumhaftes Bewußtsein（D） ………………………………………………… 98
travail de deuil（F） ……………………………………………………………… 87
treatable dementia（E） ………………………………………………………… 73
tree test（E） ……………………………………………………………………… 83
tremblement（F） ………………………………………………………………… 54
tremor（E） ………………………………………………………………………… 54
trichotillomania（E） …………………………………………………………… 85
tricyclic antidepressant（E） …………………………………………………… 37
tricyclics（E） …………………………………………………………………… 37
Trieb（D） ………………………………………………………………………… 103
Triebhandlung（D） …………………………………………………………… 103
triphasic waves（E） …………………………………………………………… 37
trouble de la conscience（F） …………………………………………………… 4
trouble mentale（F） …………………………………………………………… 59
true hallucination（E） ………………………………………………………… 54
Trugwahrnehmung（D） ……………………………………………………… 99
tuberous sclerosis（E） ………………………………………………………… 27
tubular concentric contraction（E） ………………………………………… 15
Turner syndrome（E） ………………………………………………………… 69
twilight state（E） ……………………………………………………………… 100
twin study（E） ……………………………………………………………… 66, 92

two-word sentence （E） ……………………………………………………… 80
type A behavior pattern （E） ………………………………………………… 8
typus manicus （D. v. Zerssen） （L） ……………………………………… 96
typus melancholicus （H. Tellenbach） （L） ……………………………… 99
Über-Ich （D） ……………………………………………………………… 73
Übertragung （D） …………………………………………………………… 75
Überwachheit （D） ………………………………………………………… 12
überwertige Idee （D） ……………………………………………………… 44
Übungstherapie （D） ……………………………………………………… 25
Uchida-Kraepelinscher Rechentest （D） …………………………………… 7
Umständlichkeit （D） ……………………………………………………… 7
Umzugsdepression （J. Lange） （D） ……………………………………… 88
unaided walking （E） ……………………………………………………… 88
Unbesinnlichkeit （D） ……………………………………………………… 98
unbewußt （D） ……………………………………………………………… 97
uncinate fits （H. Jackson） （E） …………………………………………… 30
unconscious （E） …………………………………………………………… 97
unconsummated marriage （E） …………………………………………… 97
undoing （E） ………………………………………………………………… 79
Uneinfühlbarkeit （D） ……………………………………………………… 15
Unfallneurose （D） ………………………………………………………… 35
Ungeschehenmachen （S. Freud） （D） …………………………………… 79
unilateral apraxia （E） ……………………………………………………… 5
unilateral spatial agnosia （E） …………………………………………… 86
unilateral spatial neglect （E） …………………………………………… 86
unipolar depression （E） …………………………………………………… 70
Unterbewußtsein （D） ……………………………………………………… 10
Unterdrückung （D） ……………………………………………………… 103
Untergrunddepression （K. Schneider） （D） …………………………… 19
Urangst （S. Freud） （D） ………………………………………………… 29
Urszene （D） ………………………………………………………………… 28
vaginismus （E） …………………………………………………………… 71
vascular dementia （E） …………………………………………………… 27
vascular depression （E） ………………………………………………… 27

vascular headache (E)	27
vegetative Neurose (D)	50
vegetative state (E)	50
Veraguthsche Falte (D)	91
Veraguth fold (E)	91
Verarmungswahn (D)	90
verbal automatism (E)	28
verbal hallucination (E)	28
verbalization (E)	28
verbal paraphasia (E)	34
verbigeration (E)	33
Verbödung (D)	32
Verdichtung (D)	1
Verdoppelungserlebnis (D)	80
Verdrängung (D)	102
Verfolgungswahn (D)	87
Vergiftungswahn (D)	88
Verhalten (D)	32
Verhältnisblödsinn (D)	103
Verlegenheitskonfabulation (D)	78
Verleugnung (D)	89
verminderte Schuldfähigkeit (D)	29
verminderte Zurechnungsfähigkeit (D)	29, 53
Verneinung (D)	89
Verneinung der Krankheit (D)	43
Verneinungswahn (D)	88
Verrücktheit (D)	94
Verschiebung (D)	9
Verschrobenheit (D)	89
Verschwendungssucht (D)	106
versive seizure (E)	94
verständlicher Zusammenhang (D)	104
verstehende Psychologie (D)	104
Verstimmtheit (D)	91

Verstimmung（D） ……………………………………………………………… 20
Versündigungswahn（D） ……………………………………………………… 35
vertigo（E） …………………………………………………………………… 11
Verwirrtheit（D） ……………………………………………………………… 36
Verwirrtheitspsychose（D） …………………………………………………… 36
verworrene Manie（D） ……………………………………………………… 36
vesania（E） …………………………………………………………………… 7
vésanie（F） …………………………………………………………………… 7
vigilance（E） ………………………………………………………………… 12
violence by partner（E） ……………………………………………………… 83
viscosity（E） ………………………………………………………………… 81
visible thoughts（E） ………………………………………………………… 31
visköses Temperament（E. Kretschmer）（D） …………………………… 81
visual agnosia（E） …………………………………………………………… 37
visual disorientation（E） …………………………………………………… 37
visual evoked potential（VEP）（E） ……………………………………… 38
visual hallucination（E） …………………………………………………… 28
visual seizure（E） …………………………………………………………… 37
visual-spatial agnosia（E） ………………………………………………… 39
visuomotor ataxia（E） ……………………………………………………… 37
vitale Depression（K. Schneider）（D） …………………………………… 57
Vitalgefühl（D） ……………………………………………………………… 57
vitalism（E） ………………………………………………………………… 57
vocal tic（E） ………………………………………………………………… 10
vocational parent（E） ……………………………………………………… 50
vollständige Remission（D） ……………………………………………… 16
voluntary admission（E） …………………………………………………… 44
voluntary guardianship system（E） ……………………………………… 81
voluntary hospitalization（E） ……………………………………………… 81
Vorbeihandeln（D） ………………………………………………………… 96
Vorbeireden（D） …………………………………………………………… 96
voyeurism（E） ……………………………………………………………… 63
vulnerability stress model（E） …………………………………………… 56
Wachanfall（D） ……………………………………………………………… 12

Wachbewußtsein（D）	12
Wachsuggestion（D）	12
Wachtraum（D）	12
Wahn（D）	99
Wahnbewußtheit（D）	99
Wahneinfall（D）	100
Wahnentwicklung（D）	100
Wahnerinnerung（D）	100
Wahngebäude（D）	99
wahnhafte Deutung（D）	100
wahnhafte Idee（D）	100
Wahnidee（D）	99
Wahninhalt（D）	100
Wahnsinn（D）	106
Wahnstimmung（D）	99
Wahnsystem（D）	99
Wahnvorstellung（D）	100
Wahnwahrnehmung（D）	100
Wandersucht（D）	83
Waschenzwang（D）	64
washing compulsion（E）	64
water intoxication（E）	97
waxy flexibility（E）	106
weak minded（E）	53
Wechsler Adult Intelligence Scale（WAIS，改訂版 WAIS-R，3版 WAIS III）（E）	7
Wechsler Intelligence Scale for Children（WISC，改訂版 WISC-R，3版 WISC III）（E）	7
Weckaminpsychose（D）	12
Weckaminvergiftung（D）	12
weekend hospital（E）	46
Weitschweifigkeit（D）	48
welfare factory for the person with mental disorder（E）	60
welfare home for the person with mental disorder（E）	60
Weltuntergangserlebnis（D）	62

Werkzeugstörung（D）	76
Wernicke aphasia（E）	7
Wernicke encephalopathy（E）	7
Wesens（ver）änderung（D）	52
West syndrome（E）	7
Widerstandanalyse（S. Freud）（D）	74
Wiedererkennung（D）	35
Wiedergutmachung（D）	74
Wiederholungszwang（D）	86
Willenlose（Psychopathen）（K. Schneider）（D）	5
Willensakt（D）	5
Willenslosigkeit（D）	5
Willensschwäche（D）	5
Wilson disease（E）	7
winter depression（E）	76
Wisconsin Card Sorting Test（WCST）（E）	7
withdrawal（E）	87, 104
Witzelsucht（D）	91
Wochenbettpsychose（D）	37
word amnesia（E）	33
word blindness（E）	34
word deafness（E）	34
word dumbness（E）	30
word finding disturbance（E）	33
word salad（E）	34
working memory（E）	36
working throuth（E）	74
World Psychiatric Association（WPA）（E）	62
Wortneubildung（D）	28
Wortrest（D）	37
Wortsalat（D）	34
Wortspielerei（D）	34
wrist-cutting（E）	104
writer's cramp（E）	50

writer's spasm (E)	50
Wunschparanoia (D)	16
Yale-Brown Obsessive Compulsive Scale (Y-BOCS) (E)	4
Yatabe-Guilford personality inventory (E)	101
Zahlenzwang (D)	26
Zählzwang (D)	26
Zahnknirschen (G)	83
Zeitbewußtsein (D)	38
Zeiterleben (D)	38
zeitliche Desorientiertheit (D)	38
Zeitlupenphänomen (D)	38
Zeitrafferphänomen (D)	38
zerebrale Kinderlähmung (D)	82
Zerfahrenheit (D)	40, 51
zirkuläre Psychose (D)	47
Zittern (D)	54
zoanthropy (E)	45
zomige Manie (D)	6
zoophilia (E)	77
zoophobia (E)	77
zoopsia (E)	77
zudeckende Methode (D)	95
Zugänglichkeit (D)	66
Zungenreden (D)	41
Zurechnungsfähigkeit (D)	19
Zurechnungsunfähigkeit (D)	19, 54
Zuspitzung der Persönlichkeit (D)	51
Zwang (D)	23
Zwangsaffekt (D)	23
Zwangsdenken (D)	23
Zwangsgreifen (D)	22
Zwangshandlung (D)	23
Zwangsidee (D)	23
Zwangslachen (D)	23

Zwangsmensch (D) ……………………………………………………………… 23
Zwangsneurose (D) ……………………………………………………………… 23
Zwangsskrupel (D) ……………………………………………………………… 23
Zwangstrieb (D) ………………………………………………………………… 23
Zwangsvorstellung (D) ………………………………………………………… 23
Zwangsweinen (D) ……………………………………………………………… 23
Zwangszeremoniell (D) ………………………………………………………… 23
Zweifelsucht (D) ………………………………………………………………… 24
Zwillingsforschung (D) ………………………………………………………… 92
Zyklothymie (D) ………………………………………………………………… 47

外国語索引 正誤表

	誤	正		誤	正
action tremor (E)	76	77	comparative psychiatry (E)	86	87
dementia (E)	80	81	double orientation (E)	79	80
endogenous (E)	78	79	flapping tremor (E)	84	85
geriatric psychiatry (E)	105	106	grasp reflex (E)	82	83
Huntington disease (E)	85	86	projective identification (M. Klein) (E)	75	76
secondary gain (E)	79	80	sekundärer Wahn (D)	79	80
spatial disorientation (E)	83	84	specific speech articulation disorder (ICD-10) (E)	77	78
subordinate (cerebral) hemisphere (E)	104	105	synchrony (E)	75	76

外 国 語 略 語 索 引

（DSM-Ⅲ, DSM-Ⅲ-R, DSM-Ⅳ, DSM-Ⅳ-TR, ICD, ICD-9, ICD-10などの出典を表わす略語は省略した。）

AA (alcoholics anonymous) ············· 2
AAMI (age-associated memory impairment) ············· 106
ADD (attention deficit disorder) ············· 71
ADEM (acute disseminated encephalomyelitis) ············· 21
ADHD (attention-deficit/hyperactivity disorder) ············· 72
AIDS dementia complex ············· 8
AGD (argy[i]rophilic grain dementia) ············· 39
ALD (adrenoleukodystrophy) ············· 91
APA (アメリカ精神医学会) ············· 60
A-T split ············· 8
BBB (blood brain barrier) ············· 26
BECCT (benign epilepsy of children with centro-temporal EEG foci) ············· 72
B-N-S Krampf (Blitz-Nick-Salaam Krampf) · 75
BPRS (Brief Psychiatric Rating Scale) ············· 14
BSE (bovine spongiform encephalopathy) ············· 7
CAT (children's apperception test) ············· 102
CBD (corticobasal degeneration) ············· 68
CIND (cognitive impairments with non dementia) ············· 102
CMI (Cornell Medical Index) ············· 34
CT (computed tomography, computerized tomography) ············· 35
DLB (dementia with Lewy bodies) ············· 105
DLBD (diffuse Lewy body disease) ············· 89
DNTC (diffuse neurofibrillary tangles with calcification) ············· 63
DQ (developmental quotient) ············· 84

DSM (Diagnostic and Statistical Manual of Mental Disorders) ············· 60
DUP (duration of untreated psychosis) ············· 61
DV (domestic violence) ············· 14
EBM (evidence-based medicine) ············· 6, 9
ECT (electroconvulsive treatment, electroconvulsive therapy) ············· 75
ED (erectile disorder) ············· 95
EE (expressed emotion) ············· 16, 30
EEG (electroencephalography) ············· 82
EEG topography ············· 82
ES (Elektroschocktherapie) ············· 75
FTD (frontotemporal dementia) ············· 64
FTD-17 (frontotemporal dementia and parkinsonism linked to chromosome 17) ············· 9
FTLD (frontotemporal lobar degeneration) ············· 64
HDS, 改定版 HDS-R (Hasegawa Dementia Scale) ············· 84
ICU psychosis (intensive care unit psychosis) ············· 46
JSPN (Japanese Society of Psychiatry and Neurology) ············· 80
KAST (Kurihama Alcoholism Screening Test) ············· 25
KFD (kinetic family drawing) ············· 77
LD (learning difficulty, learning disability) ············· 12
m-ECT (modified electroconvulsive therapy) ············· 46

MA (mental age) 60
MCI (mild cognitive impairment) 26
MEG (magnetoencephalography) 82
MLD (metachromatic leukodystrophy) 5
MMPI (Minnesota Multiphasic
　　Personality Inventory) 97
MRA (magnetic resonance angiography)
　　... 9, 38
MRI (magnetic resonance imaging) 9, 38
MRS (magnetic resonance spectroscopy)
　　... 9, 38
MS (multiple sclerosis) 69
MSA (multiple system atrophy) 69
MSLT (multiple sleep latency test) 9, 56, 80
NA (narcotics anonymous) 96
non-REM sleep 83
OKN (optokinetic nystagmus) 37
OT (occupational therapist) 36
PANSS (Positive and Negative Syndrome
　　Scale) 102
PET (positron emission tomography) 95
PIQ (performance intelligence quotient) ... 77
PML (progressive multifocal
　　leukoencephalopathy) 53
PSD (periodic synchronous discharge) 45
PSE (present state examination) 28
PSP (progressive supranuclear palsy) 53
PSW (psychiatric social worker) 61
PTSD (post-traumatic stress disorder) 55
QOL (quality of life) 57
RCT (randomized clinical trial) 98
REM (rapid eye movement) sleep 105
SANS (Scale for the Assessment of
　　Negative Symptoms) 7
SCT (sentence completion test) 93
SDAT (senile dementia of Alzheimer type) ... 3

SD-NFT (senile dementia with neurofibrillary
　　tangle) 52
SGA (second generation antipsychotics) 68
SND (striatonigral degeneration) 64
SNRI (serotonin-noradrenaline reuptake
　　inhibitor) 63
SPECT (single photon emission computed
　　tomography) 70
SSE (subacute spongiform encephalopathy)
　　... 1
SSPE (subacute sclerosing panencephalitis)
　　... 1
SSRI (selective serotonin reuptake inhibitor)
　　... 64
SST (social skills training) 44
TAT (thematic apperception test) 10
TMS (transcranial magnetic stimulation) ... 26
TIA (transient ischemic attack) 5
VEP (visual evoked potential) 38
WAIS (Wechsler Adult Intelligence Scale) ... 7
WAIS III (Wechsler Adult Intelligence
　　Scale 3 版) 7
WAIS-R (Wechsler Adult Intelligence
　　Scale 改訂版) 7
WCST (Wisconsin Card Sorting Test) 7
WHO (世界保健機構) 33
WISC (Wechsler Intelligence Scale for
　　Children) 7
WISC III (Wechsler Intelligence Scale for
　　Children 3 版) 7
WISC-R (Wechsler Intelligence Scale for
　　Children 改訂版) 7
WPA (World Psychiatric Association) 62
Y-BOCS (Yale-Brown Obsessive
　　Compulsive Scale) 4

外 国 語 略 語 索 引

(DSM-III, DSM-III-R, DSM-IV, DSM-IV-TR, ICD, ICD-9, ICD-10などの出典を表わす略語は省略した。)

AA	2	ED	95
AAMI	105	EE	16, 30
ADD	71	EEG	82
ADEM	21	EEG topography	82
ADHD	71	ES	75
AIDS dementia complex	8	FTD	64
AGD	39	FTD-17	9
ALD	91	FTLD	64
APA	60	HDS, 改定版 HDS-R	84
A-T split	8	ICU psychosis	46
BBB	26	JSPN	80
BECCT	72	KAST	25
B-N-S krampf	75	KFD	77
BPRS	14	LD	12
BSE	7	m-ECT	46
CAT	102	MA	60
CBD	68	MCI	26
CIND	102	MEG	82
CMI	34	MLD	5
CT	35	MMPI	97
DLB	105	MRA	38
DLBD	88	MRI	9, 38
DNTC	63	MRS	9, 38
DQ	84	MS	69
DSM	60	MSA	9, 69
DUP	61	MSLT	9, 56, 80
DV	14	NA	96
EBM	6, 9	non-REM sleep	82
ECT	75	OKN	37

OT	36	SPECT	70
PANSS	102	SSE	1
PET	94	SSPE	1
PIQ	77	SSRI	64
PML	53	SST	44
PSD	45	TAT	10
PSE	28	TMS	26
PSP	53	TIA	5
PSW	61	VEP	38
PTSD	55	WAIS	7
QOL	57	WAIS III	7
RCT	97	WAIS-R	7
REM sleep	105	WCST	7
SANS	7	WHO	33
SCT	93	WISC	7
SDAT	3	WISC III	7
SD-NFT	52	WISC-R	7
SGA	68	WPA	62
SND	64	Y-BOCS	4
SNRI	63		

解説用語

学習障害	learning disabiliyies（LD）（Kirk, S. L.）（E） わが国で用いられている learning disabilities（LD）という用語は米国やカナダでの用法とほぼ同一の概念である。しかし、英国では learning disabilities というと学習困難全般をさす。こうした事情もあって DSM-IV では LD に相当する読字障害、算数障害、書字表出障害を含むカテゴリーに learning disorders の用語を当てている。
職親（委託）制度	vocational parent system for intellectual dieorder 更生援護に熱意のある事業経営者を職親として、知的障害者を一定期間預け、生活指導および職業指導を委託する制度で、職業に必要な素地を与えるとともに、雇用の促進と職業における定着性を高め、福祉の向上を図ることを目的としている。その後広く精神障害者一般にも普及してきた。（英文表記は本文中を参照）
最早発痴呆（歴史用語）	dementia praecocissima（De Sanctis, S.）（L） 4歳ころまでに始まる早発性痴呆をさしたが、児童統合失調症や幼児自閉症などがクローズアップされるとともに、今日、この診断名は用いられない。
社交恐怖，社会恐怖	social phobia（DSM-III）（E） social は対人場面、社交に関することがらをあらわすもので、社会生活全般にわたる不安感を連想させる社会不安にかえて、social anxiety を社交不安、social phobia を社交恐怖とした。
循環狂気（歴史用語）	folie circulaire（F） 躁的興奮、休止、抑うつ期の3期を規則的に繰り返す精神病をさし、躁うつ病の旧概念であるが一部に緊張病などを含む。

支離滅裂	incoherence（E）, Zerfahrenheit（D）, Inkohärenz（D） ドイツ学派では、意識清明で思考がまとまらなければ滅裂（zerfahren）、意識混濁がある場合は散乱（inkohärent）という。滅裂思考（zerfahrenes Denken）は統合失調症にみられる（「精神医学辞典」より引用）。
精神作用物質	psychoactive substance（ICD-10）（E） substance-relatedなどの用語にはpsychoactiveが省略されているとみなし、精神作用物質を対応させた。
説明と承諾，インフォームド・コンセント	informed consent（E） 十分な説明を受けた上で納得しての同意なので、説明と承諾とした。
説明妄想	Erklärungswahn（D）、explanatory delusion（E） C. Wernickeが1894年に提唱した概念で二次妄想の一つ。一次的な疾病症状ではなく、幻聴、妄想などの他の精神病性症状の発生を説明するために生じた妄想をいう。
早発痴呆（歴史用語）	dementia praecox（L） 早発痴呆の概念はB. A. Morel（1856）が人生の早期（主として思春期）に発症し急速に痴呆化する一群の精神病をこの名で呼んだ。E. Kraepelin（1893）も破瓜病、緊張病、妄想性痴呆の三つの下位郡をあわせ、この早発痴呆と命名したが、E. Bleuler（1911）が早発痴呆に替わる概念としてSchizophrenieと命名した。
素行障害	conduct disorder（DSM-III）（E） DSM-IV，ICD-10の訳語では行為障害となっているが，単なる行為の障害ではなく、反復し持続する反社会的、攻撃的あるいは反抗的な行動パターンを特徴とするもので、行為障害にかえてより病態を正しく反映する素行障害（他に、行状障害、品行障害との意見もあった）をあてた。

退行期うつ病, 退行期メランコリー	involutional melancholia（E）、Involutionsmelancholie（D） E. Kraepelin が退行期精神病に記載したメランコリーは退行期うつ病の名で長く独立性が議論されたが、今日の国際分類からは除かれている。
知的障害	mental retardation（E） 精神（発達）遅滞のことであるが、行政用語ではこのように呼ぶ。
知的障害援護施設	support institutions for intellectual disorder 知的障害者の福祉では、知的障害者更生施設、知的障害者援護施設、知的障害者通勤寮、知的障害者福祉ホーム、知的障害者グループホーム、知的障害者地域ホーム、障害者福祉作業所などの施設の制度が定められている。
被害妄想, 迫害妄想, 追跡妄想	delusion of persecution（E）, Verfolgungswahn（D）, délire de persécution（F） Verfolgungswahn は被害・迫害妄想のことであるが、verfolgen（あとをつける）からわが国では長く追跡妄想の訳語を用いてきた。
恋愛妄想（病）, 被愛妄想	erotomania（E）, Liebeswahn（D）, erotomanie（G. G. de Clérambault）（F） erotomanie には、他人から愛されている妄想内容と、恋愛妄想を主題とする妄想性障害の2つの用法がある。
ワーンジン, 妄覚錯乱（歴史用語）	Wahnsinn（D） Wahnsinn は、一般のドイツ語では、精神異常、狂気をいう。W. Griesinger、H. Neumann、C. Wernicke、E. Kraepelin らの用い方によると、比較的急性に発症し、幻覚、被害妄想、不安を主症状とし、意識は概ね清明な状態を指す。呉秀三は、"わーんじん"と表記し、石田昇は、妄想あるいは妄想病としている。日独ともに古い概念であるが、単なる錯乱 Verwirrtheit と区別して、妄覚錯乱の名称を提唱する。

歴 史 用 語

ウェザニア	vesania（E），vésanie（F）
共生幼児精神病	symbiotic infantile psychosis（M. Mahler）（E）
疑惑狂	folie de dout（F）
交代狂気	folie alterne（F）
最早発痴呆	dementia praecocissima（De Sanctis）（L）
循環狂気	folie circulaire（F）
循環精神病	zirkuläre Psychose（D）
シルダー病	Schilder disease（E）
振戦麻痺	paralysis agitans（L）
精神乖離症	schizophrenia（E）
精神薄弱	mental deficiency, oligophrenia（E），Schwachsinn（D），arriération mentale（F）
精神分裂	Schizophrenia（E）
精神分裂症	Schizophrenia（E）
精神分裂病→統合失調症	Schizophrenia（E）
早発痴呆	dementia praecox（L）
単純痴呆	dementia simplex（L）
てんかん病質	epileptoid（E），Epileptoid（D）
動物磁気，生動磁気	magnétisme animal（F），animal magnetism（E）
ヒステロエピレプシー	hysteroepilepsy（E）
フェニル焦性ぶどう酸精神薄弱	oligophrenia phenylpyruvica（L）
不統一狂気	folie discordante（P. Chaslin）（F）
変質	dégénérescence（Morel, B. A.）（F），degeneration（E），Entartung（D）
偏執狂	Verrücktheit（D）
麻痺（性）痴呆	dementia paralytica（L）
メランコリーの激越発作，憂うつ激昂［高］	raptus melancholicus（L）
妄想（性）痴呆	dementia paranoides（L）
幼年痴呆	dementia infantilis（T. Heller）（L）
らい恐怖（症）	lepraphobia（E）
利口ぶり阿呆，釣り合い阿呆	Verhältnisblödsinn（D），démence relative（F）

理性的狂気	folie raisonnante（F）
リペマニー	lypémanie（E. Esquirol）（F）
類てんかん性格	epileptoid personality（E）
ワーンジン，妄覚錯乱	Wahnsinn（D）

人 名 索 引

(ファミリーネームを先頭に出してアルファベット順に配列した。)
人名のあとの数字は本文のページ数を表わす。

Adler, A. ……………………………… 17	Ellenberger, H. F. ……………………… 66
Arieti, S. ……………………………… 56	Enke, W. ……………………………… 81
Asperger, H. ………………………… 44	Erikson, E. H. ………………… 20, 38, 75
Baillarger, J. ………………………… 58	Esquirol, E. ……………………… 100, 104
Balint, M. ………………………… 19, 37	Ey, H. …………………………………… 18
Ballet, G. ……………………………… 96	Fail, G. ………………………………… 12
Bateson, G. ………………………… 69, 80	Falret, J-P. …………………………… 47
Berne, E. ……………………………… 33	Federn, P. …………………………… 37
Birnbaum, K. ……………………… 31, 89	Flournoy, T. ………………………… 64
Blankenburg, W. …………………… 41	Frank, R. T. ………………………… 27
Bleuler, E. ……………………… 18, 87, 91	Frankl, V. E. ………………………… 106
Bleuler, M. ……………………… 79, 81, 208	Freeman, W. ………………………… 65
Bonhoeffer, K. …………………… 10, 14	Freud, S. ……… 7, 8, 11, 28, 29, 74, 78, 90
Bürger-Prinz, H. …………………… 81	Fromm=Reichmann, F. …………… 77
Cairns, H. …………………………… 98	Geschwind, N. ……………………… 13
Capgras, J. ………………………… 8, 10	Gibbs, E. L. ……………………… 49, 75
Ceillier, A. …………………………… 86	Gibbs, F. A. ……………………… 49, 75
Charcot, J. M. ……………………… 68	Goldstein, K. ………………… 72, 83, 85
Chaslin, P. ………………………… 29, 91	Griesinger, W. ……………………… 70, 209
Claude, H. …………………………… 104	Guiraud, P. …………………………… 11
Clérambault, G. G. de … 59, 81, 105, 209	Häfner, H. …………………………… 42
Conrad, K. …………………………… 9	Halbey, K. …………………………… 31
Cotard, J ……………………………… 34	Hecker, E. …………………………… 83
Courbon, P. ………………………… 12	Heller, T. …………………………… 102
Cramer, H. …………………………… 24	Huber, G. ………………………… 47, 67
Delay, J. ……………………………… 44	藤縄昭 ………………………………… 38
De Sanctis, S. …………………… 35, 207	Husserl, E. …………………………… 72
Dewhurst, K. ………………………… 9	井村恒郎 ……………………………… 33
Dupré, E. ………………………… 24, 25	Jackson, H. ……………… 11, 30, 51, 98
Ekbom, K. A. ………………………… 88	Jaensch, E. R. ……………………… 73

Janet, P. ……………………… 25, 28, 55, 60	森田正馬 ……………………… 19, 52, 88
Janz, D. ……… 12, 30, 32, 48, 56, 63, 91	Morita, M. ……………………………… 52
Jaspers, K. ……………………………… 6	Neumann, H. ……………………… 70, 209
Jung, C. G. ………………… 6, 22, 28, 92	岡上和雄 ………………………………… 50
Kahlbaum, L. ………………………… 104	Otto, R. ………………………………… 81
Kanner, L. ……………………………… 65	Penfield, W. …………………………… 61
Kassanin, J. …………………………… 76	Pick, A. ………………………………… 46
Kernberg, O. ………………………… 22	Reboul-Lachaux, J. ……………………… 8
Kielholz, P. …………………………… 49	Régis, E. ……………………………… 97
Kirk, S. L. …………………………… 207	Rogers, C. R. ………………………… 103
Klein, M. …………………………… 74, 75	Roth, M. ………………………………… 71
Kleist, K. ……………………………… 93	Rümke, H. C. ………………………… 92
小林八郎 ………………………………… 57	Sakel, M ………………………………… 6
古澤平作 ………………………………… 1	Schneider, K. ……… 5, 13, 19, 20, 22, 28, 41,
Kraepelin, E. ……………… 26, 66, 208, 209	48, 49, 55, 57, 61, 83, 84, 98, 102
Kretschmer, E. · 12, 13, 42, 68, 81, 89, 92	Schulte, W. …………………………… 79
Lacan, J. ……………………… 22, 28, 66	Schultz, J. H. ………… 5, 51, 65, 72, 93
Lange, J. ……………………………… 88, 101	Séglas, J. ……………………………… 28
Langfeldt, G. ………………………… 76	Selye, H. ……………………………… 86
Lennox, W. G. ………………………… 61	Semon, R. ……………………………… 17
Leonhard, K. …………………………… 90	Sérieux, P. ……………………………… 10
Lhermitte, J. …………………………… 72	下田光造 ………………………………… 46
Lidz, T. ………………………………… 90	Sommer, M. ………………………… 51, 71
Mahler, M. …………………………… 22	Spitz, R ………………………………… 5
Masterson, J. F. ……………………… 97	Stauder, K. H. ………………………… 70
Mayer-Gross, W. …………………… 28, 97	Störring, G. …………………………… 31
Meduna, L. J. ………………………… 97	Stransky, E. ………………………… 55, 70
Menninger, K. ………………………… 96	Sullivan, H. S. ………………… 16, 64, 85
Meyer, A. ……………………………… 60	Szondi, L. ……………………………… 8
Minkowski, E. ……… 29, 89, 95, 101	Tellenbach, H. ………………………… 98
三宅鑛一 ………………………………… 97	Todd, J. ………………………………… 9
Monakow, C. v. ……………………… 74	Tramer, M. …………………………… 64
Moniz, E. ……………………………… 65	Tulving, E. …………………………… 9
Morel, B. A. ………………………… 93, 208	臺弘 …………………………………… 50, 57
Moreno, J. L. ………………………… 44, 55	Watts, J. W. …………………………… 65
Morlaas, J. …………………………… 48	Waxman, S. G. ………………………… 13

Weitbrecht, H. J. ·································· 79
Weizsäcker, V. v. ································ 19
Wernicke, C. ························ 8, 10, 27, 54,
                                     63, 79, 208, 209
Weygandt, W. ································· 34

Wieck, H. H. ····································· 73
Winkler, W. Th. ································· 38
Wynne, L. ·· 19
Zerssen, D. v. ····································· 96

参 考 資 料

ICD-10 精神および行動の障害 DCR 研究用診断基準．中根允文他訳．医学書院．1994
ICD-10 精神および行動の障害―臨床記述と診断ガイドライン―（新訂版）．監訳 融道男他．医学書院．2005
APA 精神医学用語集．加藤伸勝監訳．医学書院．1986
心のケアのためのカウンセリング大事典．松原達哉共編．培風館．2005
新版精神医学事典．編者代表加藤正明．弘文堂．1993
精神神経学用語集．日本精神神経学会精神神経学用語委員会編．社団法人日本精神神経学会．1989
精神医学事典増補版．加藤正明他編集．弘文堂．2001
精神医学大事典．新福尚武編．講談社．1984
精神分析事典．編集代表小此木啓吾，岩崎学術出版社．2002
神経学用語集．日本神経学会用語委員会編．文光堂．1993
心身症用語集．社団法人日本心身医学会用語委員会編．医学書院．1999
睡眠障害国際分類診断とコードの手引き．日本睡眠学会診断分類委員会訳．1994
睡眠障害の対応と治療ガイドライン．睡眠障害の診断・治療ガイドライン研究会（内山真）編．じほう．2002
DSM-IV-TR 精神疾患の分類と診断の手引き新訂版．高橋三郎他訳．医学書院．2005
てんかん学会用語集．日本てんかん学会用語委員会編．2004
メンタルヘルスハンドブック．上里一郎他監修．同朋舎出版．1989
臨床心理大辞典[改訂版]．氏原寛共編．培風館．2004

以　上

おわりに

　2006年度に「統合失調症関連用語」および「痴呆（症）関連用語」補遺を理事会、評議員会の承認を得て本学会ホームページに掲載した。翌2007年度に用語集本文の全面的改訂を行い今後の多少の修正を含めて基本的に改訂版原案を理事会、評議員会で承認して頂き同じく本学会のホームページに掲載し、広く一般会員からの意見を求めた。その結果2007年8月末日までに寄せられた意見を当委員会で検討して多少の訂正を加え理事会で承認されたものが本用語集である。この3年間で計28回の委員会を開催した（議事録はすべて学会誌に掲載）。近年の新用語の増加に伴い本用語集は旧版に比べほぼ倍量になった。この間の作業はかなり大変な分量で本委員会委員およびオブザーバーの各位には、遠路の方もおられ、多大の時間と労力を費やし並々ならぬ情熱をもって夜遅くまで議論して頂いた。そのため学会事務局の方々には随分ご迷惑をかけた。私自身も相当時間を取られたがその苦労よりも大変勉強になり、また楽しくもあった。

　ここに曲がりなりにも本用語集が出版の運びにまで至ったのはひとえにこれらの方々のご尽力の賜物であり、委員長として深く感謝している。また、常に暖かく見守り適切な支援と助言と頂いた理事長はじめ各理事および評議員の方々、更には多くの会員諸氏に心から御礼申し上げたい。とはいっても本用語集は一通過点に過ぎない。冒頭にも指摘したように今後更に充実したものにするためには、従来のように長い年月をおかず、2, 3年毎に点検し修正、補足していく必要がある。そのため本委員会は（メンバーは変わるとしても）継続して活動してゆく必要があり、引き続いて理事・評議員各位および一般会員の方々の一層のご指導、御協力をお願いする次第である。

　2008年春

松下昌雄

© 2008　　　　　　　　　　　　　　　　　　　　2008年6月17日発行

精神神経学用語集　改訂6版

（定価はカバーに表示してあります）

編　集　日本精神神経学会・精神科用語検討委員会

発行者　服部 治夫

検印省略

印　刷　株式会社 藤美社

株式会社 新興医学出版社
〒113-0033　東京都文京区本郷6-26-8
電話　03(3816)2853　　振替口座　00120-8-191625

ISBN978-4-88002-681-7